Language Disorders in Children

Language Disorders in Children

A RESOURCE BOOK FOR
SPEECH/LANGUAGE PATHOLOGISTS

By

MERLIN J. MECHAM, Ph.D.

Professor
Speech Pathology and Audiology
University of Utah
Salt Lake City, Utah

and

MARY LOUISE WILLBRAND, Ph.D.

Director
Speech Pathology and Audiology
University of Utah
Salt Lake City, Utah

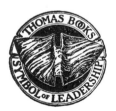

CHARLES C THOMAS · PUBLISHER
Springfield · Illinois · U.S.A.

Published and Distributed Throughout the World by

CHARLES C THOMAS • PUBLISHER

Bannerstone House

301-327 East Lawrence Avenue, Springfield, Illinois, U.S.A.

© *1979, by* CHARLES C THOMAS • PUBLISHER

ISBN 0-398-03865-1

Library of Congress Catalog Card Number: 78-10777

With THOMAS BOOKS careful attention is given to all details of manufacturing and design. It is the Publisher's desire to present books that are satisfactory as to their physical qualities and artistic possibilities and appropriate for their particular use. THOMAS BOOKS will be true to those laws of quality that assure a good name and good will.

Library of Congress Cataloging in Publication Data

Mecham, Merlin J.
    Language disorders in children.

    Bibliography: p.
    Includes index.
    1. Speech disorders in children. 2. Children—
Language. I. Willbrand, Mary Louise, joint author.
II. Title.
RJ496.S7M42   618.9′28′55   78-10777
ISBN 0-398-03865-1

Printed in the United States of America

C-1

PREFACE

During the past decade there have been dynamic changes in the concepts related to child language acquisition. The mechanistic theory of Skinner lost much of its impact under the heavy influence of Chomsky's theory that an innate capacity for language acquisition enables the individual to formulate his own grammar in the face of an impoverished environment. This latter theory, along with Chomsky's theory of generative grammar, has stimulated a renaissance in the study of language acquisition. Expanding linguistic theories of syntax, semantics, phonology, and pragmatics are continuously displaying an impact on the study of children's language. Likewise, utilization of piagetian philosophy in the study of cognition and new growth in the study of verbal information processing have stimulated new interest in the application of these developments to the field of speech pathology.

The electrifying effects of all three of these fields (linguistic theory, cognitive psychology, and perception) have resulted in a proliferation of literature, mainly in the form of collections of chapters by large numbers of authors in anthology-like volumes. It is becoming progressively more difficult and frustrating for speech pathologists to try to keep abreast of this literature and to apply the current information available to the clinical population.

The authors of this book feel that there is a need to present various views representing the present state-of-the-art and to furnish some direction to the study of current literature that should prove useful to both the college classroom and direct clinical applications. This book should serve well as a resource book for practicing speech pathologists and graduate students in the field of speech pathology.

However, this book is not intended merely to rehash already presented materials. In addition to presenting issues and suggest-

v

ing solutions, all sections contain expressions of the biases of the authors. These biases are presented without apology and are clearly designated as reflecting our own interpretations.

Chapter 1 describes patterns, contexts, and expectations in the course of a child's normal development of language; it presents linguistic foundations and contemporary developmental issues. Some verbal information processing correlates to language development are analyzed. Chapter 2 discusses various disorders of language among children and includes descriptions of cognitive, semantic, syntactic, phonological, and pragmatic disorders. Chapters 3 and 4 summarize formal and informal testing procedures for identification, placement, and assessment of progress relative to language intervention. Chapter 5 discusses intervention strategies for minimally handicapped children with language disorders; Chapter 6 presents intervention strategies for severely and/ or multiply handicapped children with language disorders. The two chapters on diagnosis and the two chapters on treatment are interdependent.

We acknowledge with special thanks suggestions made by Jon Eisenson, who kindly consented to read portions of the manuscript. Special recognition goes to Blanche Buchanan, who typed and retyped the manuscripts. We are also indebted to many of our colleagues and students who have contributed in one way or another. We especially thank our dear families who have been so patient and encouraging.

M.J.M.
M.L.W.

CONTENTS

Language Disorders in Children

Chapter 1

NORMATIVE ASPECTS OF LANGUAGE AND LANGUAGE DEVELOPMENT

THE CHILD'S LINGUISTIC FOUNDATIONS

O STENSIBLY, THIS BOOK deals with evaluation and intervention procedures for the speech pathologist working with language disorders in children. However, in any practical approach to evaluation or intervention, there must be available some standard against which discrepancies may be evaluated and objectives may be operationally defined. Such a standard may be found in the normal patterns of language.

The present section gives descriptions of the developed patterns of language. The descriptions are admittedly brief and heavily slanted toward transformation and generative grammar theory; they are documented extensively enough to enable a student or clinician to pursue any of the concepts in greater detail.

Verbal language can be classified into six symbolic behavioral processes: (1) semantic decoding, (2) syntactic decoding, (3) phonological decoding, (4) semantic encoding, (5) syntactic encoding, and (6) phonological encoding. That we utilize semantics, syntax, and phonology in linguistic encoding or decoding seems to be clear. However, it is not so clear whether these components of the linguistic system are decoded and encoded sequentially or simultaneously during the communicative process. One of the components may be in error while the others are accurate. How many times have you said a sentence that was syntactically and phonologically grammatical but as soon as it was uttered you said, "that's not what I mean. I mean . . ." and a new sentence emerged. Of course, to assume that the speaker is always most concerned with the semantic component seems naive.

Additionally, words, phrases, and sentences have different meanings depending on the situation. A listener may need to know the situation to interpret the message. Suppose a college student calls home and says, "I had to see Dr. Brown today." The

3

parent responds, "My goodness, what's wrong?" A long discussion and a great deal of confusion may result if the student means Dr. Brown is a professor, the parent interprets Dr. Brown to be a physician and/or the parent says, "What's wrong?" to indicate "Are you ill?" the student interprets "What's wrong?" to mean, "Are you having trouble with the course?" or "Did you have a personal problem?" or "Did Dr. Brown think something was wrong?" Situations such as this one expand the linguistic variables by pragmatics.

The complicated and involved sequence in processing language will be interpreted differently by various authors, and still much of it will depend on speculation. It seems sufficient to say that the components of language (semantics, syntax, and phonology) are interwoven in the encoding and decoding process. The communicative act will also be affected by the relationship of the speakers and the propositions, performatives, and presuppositions governing the use of language in social contexts (pragmatics).

The components of language semantics (meaning), syntax (word + word), and phonology (sound and sound sequencing) are represented in the whole linguistic system.

The following simple schematic representation may clarify the relationship of the components of language.

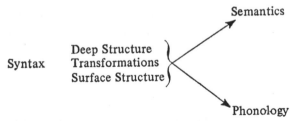

This drawing would represent syntax as the central factor in three interrelated components.*

The following discussion shows how each of these components can be further broken down into more detailed descriptions.

---

* The relationship of the components of language is currently open for considerable discussion and debate. We recognize the movement in the 1970s toward greater emphasis of semantics, and at the same time maintain that until more is known about semantics this conservative perspective concerning the centrality of syntax is warranted—certainly in the description and treatment of language problems in children.

The morpheme is the smallest meaningful unit of grammar. One or more morphemes may compose a word. Free morphemes are words. *Boy, run,* and *happy* are free morphemes. Bound morphemes include all other minimal units and may be added to a free morpheme. Thus *s* is a bound morpheme that may have various semantic interpretations. The most common interpretation is the plural. Other bound morphemes may be *un, ness, re, by, ed,* etc.

The lexicon of language is a "dictionary" of morphemes. The lexicon, as well as language as a whole, contains the components of semantics, syntax, and phonology. As words enter the lexicon the phonological representation of the word is noted—the syntax is provided in terms of category of the word, i.e. noun, verb, adjective, determiner, etc. and where this word may appear in a sequence of word order, such as before a verb phrase (. . . .VP) or after a determiner (det. . . . .)—and abstract semantic markers, in the form of binary semantic features, are attached. For nouns, the binary features include basic markers such as ± common, ± animate, and ± human, as well as necessary bits of information such as ± male and ± married. The list may be expanded as far as necessary to include pertinent information.

A lexicon and a set of rewrite rules comprise the base structure of language. What is structure? Structure or the syntax of language is represented by a hierarchical order of rules. From most abstract to least abstract these levels are deep, base, or underlying structure; transformation; and surface structure.

These rules, which are continuously being evolved by linguists, are presented in terms of a grammar. Generative grammar, a theoretical model initially proposed by Noam Chomsky (1957, 1965), is an idealized set of finite rules that can account for the infinite number of grammatical sentences and none of the ungrammatical sentences of a language. Branching tree diagrams are often used by the linguist as formal representations of the hierarchical structure of a sentence. These representations are called phrase markers and they use symbols to represent the constituents of a sentence.

An example of the formal representation of the branching tree diagram follows:

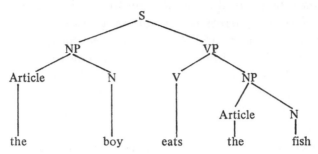

A series of these tree diagrams are used to indicate different levels of structure as well as structural changes. Imagine a series of these trees with the syntactic and semantic subclassification specified represented by this schematic diagram:

S
△ - - - - - - - - - - - - - - - - - - deep structure

S
△ - - - - - - - - - - - - - - - - modified structure

S
△ - - - - - - - - - - - - - - - - modified structure

S
△ - - - - - - - - - - - - - - - - modified structure

S
△ - - - - - - - - - - - - - - - surface structure

The following discussion may help explain what we have represented by these figures.

The symbols may be class (or category) symbols such as S (sentence), NP (noun phrase) or VP (verb phrase); they may be lexical symbols such as *the, boy,* or *eats,* or they may be cover symbols such as X, used to represent any string in the grammar. The plus sign (+) is often used to represent concatenation of the symbols. Therefore, among many possibilities, simple strings could be S + S, NP + VP, the + boy + eats, or X + S + VP.

These symbols are used in the syntactical component to represent the three levels of hierarchical structure. The grammatical features of language govern the hierarchical arrangements of various constituents in the sentence. Grammatical rules designate relationships (and relate two parallel structures; *s* relates two sentences in S → S + and + S; order indicates subject-object relationship, etc.); classification is also designated (ball is a noun, etc.), as well as syntactic meanings of plurality *(s)*, possession *('s)*, and tense *(will, did)*. Syntactic markers are governed by those rules that apply to arrangements between words, and morphological markers are governed by rules that apply to arrangements of morphemes (stem words, affixes, etc. within words).

The base or underlying structure of the syntactical component is composed of a set of rewrite rules and a lexicon. The rewrite rules specify the basic grammatical relationships, such as S → NP + VP. The lexicon specifies the phonological representation of the words and the syntactic features and the semantic markers for the lexical categories.

The next level consists of the transformational rules. Transformations are rules that map deep structure into surface structure. The transformational rules of a grammar apply to the phrase marker rather than to the vocabulary string. Transformations may be optional or obligatory and describe how symbols may be rearranged, added to, deleted, or substituted. Thus, in addition to a base structure, a grammar contains a transformational structure and the surface structure is determined by applications of transformations.

Surface structures are the final derived phrase markers of the syntactic component of a grammar. They are the least abstract and present a structural description of the sentence that we hear or speak.

Jacobs and Rosenbaum (1968, p. 57) have suggested a formula that represents the basic *nesting* rules by which base sentence strings are generated.

$$S \rightarrow NP + Aux + VP$$

$$NP \rightarrow \begin{Bmatrix} NP + S \\ \text{or} \\ N(P) + (S) \end{Bmatrix}$$

$$VP \rightarrow VB + (NP) + \begin{Bmatrix} (NP) \\ \text{or} \\ (S) \end{Bmatrix}$$

This base structure is interpreted by the semantic component.

The conventions used are defined as follows: S = sentence; NP = noun phrase (a noun phrase that contains a preposition is written PP); VP = verb phrase; → = is written as; VB = verb; ( ) = optional segment; and {} = a choice of upper or lower string of segments.

It can be seen that the number of basic strings is probably finite but that an infinite number of surface sentences could be generated by the use of transformations such as substitution, conjunction, or transposition.

1. N + Aux + VB
   Johnnie can write.
2. NP + Aux + VB
   The dog can bite.
3. N + Aux + VB + N
   People can eat meat.
4. NP + Aux + VB + N
   The dog can bite children.
5. N + Aux + VB + N + PP
   Fish can lay eggs in the sand.
6. NP + [N + Aux + VB +]* Aux + VB
   The dog that can bite has died.
7. NP + Aux + VB + N + PP
   The dog can bite children on the leg.
8. N + Aux + VB + [N + Aux + VB + PP]
   Mother does hope we can go with her.
9. NP + Aux + VB + [N + Aux + VB + NP]
   The teacher could tell you had hurt your leg.
10. NP + [N + Aux + VB] + Aux + VB + NP
    The dog that can bite has taken the bone.
11. N + Aux + VB + N + [N + Aux + VB + NP]
    Mother will tell sister she may tend the baby.
12. NP + Aux + VB + NP + [N + Aux + VB + NP]
    The teacher has told the children they should go home.
13. NP + [N + Aux + VB + N] + Aux + VB + NP + PP

---

* Brackets represent embedded sentences. Embedded sentences may be introduced by an embedded sentence marker such as *that, when, which,* etc., but frequently such marker words do not appear.

The dog that could bite us has buried a bone in the
ground.
14. NP + [N + Aux + VB + N] + Aux + VB + NP +
[N + Aux + VB + N + NP]
The lady that will teach us has told our principal she will
give us a test.

The features that mark the relationship between symbolic
units and the aspects of reality being represented by them are
called *semantic* features. Meanings of the various constituents
of a sentence are combined in such a way as to result in a meaning for the entire sentence, i.e. the meaning of combined words
results in sentence semantics (Cazden, 1971). Sentence meanings
are likewise combined in such a way as to result in concept meaning, etc. However, semantics may extend beyond the limits of
syntax. In other words, the relevant factor in semantics may be
the way in which the speaker-hearer views the world. Thus, while
semantics extends beyond a sentence into the meaning of a message, or the various meanings, depending on a situation, semantics may also vary individually. Individual semantic interpretations are particularly apparent in child language.

Theoretically, the surface structure is interpreted by the
phonological component for the pronunciation of the sentence.
Phonological features of language are the basic psychoacoustic
elements that serve as brick and mortar out of which various elements of language are made. Phonology includes perceptual
boundaries of the sound spectrum labeled "phonemes" and also
the prosodic aspects of speech having to do with stress contours,
etc. (For greater detail on the phonological characteristics of the
English language, see Chomsky and Halle, 1968.)

Culture-Sensitive Variations

Culture-sensitive variations of oral language cannot be generalized except within the bounds of the particular culture in question since they likely are heavily influenced by that culture. Although the existence of the following phenomena is universal,
the particular forms in which they appear vary considerably
from culture to culture (for example, see Kessler, 1971 for com-

parison of English and Italian). These *forms* are referred to as culture-sensitive aspects of language. They include, among other things, transformational rules, morphological rules, and phonological rules. The latter set of rules is probably more easily affected by shadings of environmental or cultural differences than the others since languages all have various intralanguage dialects in which stress tendencies seem to play a predominant role.

There are undoubtedly other specific culturally determined language phenomena that could be included, but the aforementioned ones are presented here as illustrative. They will be briefly described in terms of American English.

Transformations

Grammatical deviations from the basic phrase structures (described above) are considered to be syntactic transformations. The forms of transformations, like the form of words, differ greatly from one language culture to another but are normally rather uniform within a given language culture. We therefore cannot talk about universal transformations. Some of the more common transformations found in the American culture (Jacobs and Rosenbaum, 1968) include the following: (1) The imperative transformation, which implies that the subject "you" is always understood but may be omitted from surface structure. (2) The question form of the sentence, the rules for which imply that the interrogative form (answered by yes or no) moves the auxiliary to the front of the subject noun phrase and the question form (which requires more than a yes or no answer) places the *wh* word* at the beginning of the sentence, followed by the interrogative form. (3) The negation transformation form of the sentence, the rules for which are rather complex, but a simple rule is the introduction of the deep structure constituent into surface structure by use of no or not. (4) The modification form of the sentence, the rules of which imply that the so-called adjective and/or adverb modifiers† can be used in pre-verb-phrase positions even though technically they are parts of the

---

* *Wh* words are words such as what, where, when, who, how, etc.

† Adjectives are probably nonverb verbals (Jacobs and Rosenbaum, 1968, p. 65).

verb phrase. (5) The possessive form of the sentence, the rules of which imply that the subject noun be inflected by an /'s/ as a substitute for the relative clause, e.g. "the book that belongs to John" becomes "John's book." (6) Prepositional transformation implies that the preposition is a deep feature of the verb but is introduced into surface structure through closed-class-words. (7) The adverb and/or particle transformations, the rules for which imply that adverbs and particles are deep features of the verb but are introduced into surface structure as words separate from the verb (some surface words can serve as either prepositions or particles, e.g. up, over, but their syntactic functions differ). (8) The contraction transformation, the rules of which, simply stated, imply that a single word, such as is, can be assimilated into another word by the addition of a lesser number of phonemes, such as /s/ (e.g. "it is" becomes "it's"), or that several words, such as man, woman, child, etc., can be replaced by a reduced number of words, such as they. (9) Passive transformation, the rule for which reverses the position of the subject and object and inserts the preposition by before the subject noun phrase.

There are many other transformations, but those mentioned above are rather stable among persons in speaking American English. The rules for American English transformations do not necessarily correspond with the rules of other languages serving similar functions.

Morphology and Phonology

Morphological change for grammatical agreement is an interlanguage universal, but the specific forms of the morphological changes differ drastically from one language to another. Some of the inflectional changes in American English include the following: (1) Number agreement, in which the form of the noun indicates whether it represents a plural or a singular concept, and in which the form of the verb changes to agree in number with its subject nouns. (2) Tense agreement, in which the auxiliary agrees with the concept of point in time and in which the verb agrees with the auxiliary in reflecting tense concept. (3) Genitive agreement, in which the noun form agrees with the deep meaning of possession. (4) Person agreement, in which the pronoun agrees with the deep structure person concept and the verb agrees, within certain tense restrictions, with the pronoun in reflecting person. (5) The auxiliary-handling in surface structure, in which it is either omitted, included as a separate word, or assimilated into the verb, e.g. "bird does fly" becomes "bird flies." (6) Negation agreement, in which a negative concept of a statement is reflected by the appearance of such grammatical markers as *un* (unbutton), *non,* etc.

There are undoubtedly other inflectional word changes important to American English, but those listed above are ones that often create difficulty in children with learning or language disorders.

The phonemic structure of words is an arbitrary and socially determined phenomena that seems to be constantly undergoing slight changes. There is a tendency for members of a given social region to use that system of segmental forms in words with which they have the closest and most frequent contact. In American English, the written form of the English vocabulary is uniform over the country and is fairly similar to that used by the rest of the English-speaking world. The phonemic forms of spoken words however vary slightly as a function of group isolations that are created by some type of geographical or social barrier. Changes resulting from geographical barriers have made spoken American English sound different from the English spoken in Great Britain, Australia, etc.; such differences are called accents and are primarily the result of stress and vowel changes that seem to be highly vulnerable to environmental influences. Dialectal differences within the United States seem also to be mainly differences in stress and vowel changes (subcultural dialects and other variations are discussed in another section of this chapter).

A thorough discussion of rules for phonological stress contours can be found in Chomsky and Halle (1968). A general, but unrefined description of these rules as they apply to simple verbs, nouns, and adjectives is given below mainly to illustrate that stress in English is governed by socially determined rules rather than being "inherent in the phonological matrix of the lexical entry" (p. 66).

1. Main Stress Rule

Verbs: Primary stress is placed on the penultimate syllable in the absence of a strong cluster in the word; if one or more strong clusters (i.e. tense, vowel, or lax vowel followed by two or more consonants) are present, the primary stress is placed upon the final strong cluster (pp. 70-71).

Nouns: Primary stress is generally placed upon the syllable with the strong cluster or upon the penultimate vowel in the absence of a strong cluster—lax vowels found at the end of nouns are disregarded; such lax vowels may or may not be followed by a single consonant (p. 72).

Adjectives: The main stress rules apply to adjectives approximately the same as they do to nouns and verbs.

2. Alternating Stress and Stress Adjustment Rules

In a large majority of nouns, verbs, and adjectives with three or more syllables, the primary stress is on the antepenultimate vowel. This is termed the alternating stress rule. The stress adjustment rule requires that, within a word, all nonprimary stresses are weakened by one. Therefore, in words having a strong cluster at the end but having three or more syllables, the primary stress is on the antepenultimate syllable and the final cluster receives tertiary stress through the influence of the alternating stress and stress adjustment rules (p. 77).

3. Nuclear Stress and Compound Rules

The nuclear stress rule requires that where there are a series of primary stresses in a sentence or phrase, the final stress gets the nuclear heavy stress and all other stresses are reduced by one (p. 90). The compound stress rule, on the other hand, assigns primary stress to the first of two stress peaks in compound word construction, such as chemistry laboratory, the heavy stress is given to the first of the two heavy stress peaks rather than to the last (p. 92).

The above stress rules are presented as cultural-specific aspects after the recommendation by Chomsky and Halle (1968, pp. 43-44) that they are in large part rather specific to American English grammar. These rules are accompanied by specific vowel change rules that have been described in some detail by Chomsky and Halle; a major change in the vowel, for example, is a shift from tense to lax or to neutral whenever the primary stress is reduced to a lesser level.

Subcultural Variations

As mentioned previously, cultural-specific aspects of oral language behavior are learned through social imitation and may change rapidly within the subcultures of a single language culture. Regional dialects and "common" versus "cultured" speech differences have developed as a result of this tendency. Also the influence of a primarily foreign language upon the use of English as a second language has resulted in different characteristics of English as used by the American blacks, Spanish Americans, native Americans, etc.

Dialectal Variations

Because of variations in topography, settlement history, types of interrelationships, etc., dialect regions are often difficult to delimit (Gleason, 1961, p. 403). However, in America there are three major dialectal areas commonly referred to as northern, midland, and southern. Each of these are comprised of a group of subdialects; and thus it is fallacious to speak of any area as having only a single dialect. The sharpest boundary seems to be found along the Virginia Blue Ridge Mountains—separating rather sharply the midland from the southern group in the East (Gleason, 1961, p. 403). Also large cities, such as Chicago, New York, Detroit, and Washington, D.C., tend to evolve some of their own dialectal and subgroup variations.

The dialectal differences are primarily phonemic and phonetic such as the New England's pronunciation of /aw/ being often pronounced as /æw/ in the South, or the New York City pronunciation of the /ð/ as a dental stop whereas it is pronounced as a dental fricative by non-New Yorkers. The tendency for omitting the pronunciation of the /r/ before other consonants or at the end of words by people in eastern New England, in New York City, and in the South is another example. There are also some analogic differences in dialect that are not as regular as the phonemic (Gleason, 1961, p. 404). An example of this is the southern use of "halp" as the past tense of "help."

As the geographical barriers become less pronounced because of improved travel and mass communication facilities (television), the regional variations have gradually become somewhat less distinct. However, the child from a poor southern or south midland background, who is transferred into a northern urban environment, may still suffer from both his and the teacher's lack of knowledge or understanding of the dialectal differences. His tendency to simplify consonant clusters and differences in vowel pronunciations may create difficulty for him. His variations in stress and vowel shifts as well as in transformational forms may create additional stress between him and his northern peers.

Class differences do not seem to effect pronunciations so much within a given region, but transformations and vocabulary of the lower socioeconomic class may be different. The lower class's skills with language center more around descriptions of concrete and emotional experiences than around abstract operational planning; the vocabulary is more concrete and more closely bound to sensory-motor imagery (Riessman, 1962).

Pidginization and Creolization

Pidginization of a language occurs in a minority group whose native language is different from that of the dominant language; the vocabulary is selected from the dominant language, but the syntax and phonology are heavily influenced by the minority group's native language. "If a pidgin language becomes the native language for a group of speakers, it is said to be creolized" (Taylor, 1971, p. 20).

CREOLIZATION. In the case of black American English, the pidginizations, which occurred in the early history of the use of English by the blacks, eventually became creolized when they lost their original native languages. There are some variations in black English that should be of importance in our understanding minority group differences in language. Variations in black American speech are so widespread and stereotyped that their speech patterns are considered to be different, even though the majority of their patterns are the same as their white American peers. Such differences are apparently great enough to create some social barriers and also to interfere with "appropriate" educational success. Black children in American urban ghetto schools are noted for their generalized failure in the mastery of reading skills. "The most important [instances] are those in which large-scale phonological differences coincide with important grammatical differences. The result of this coincidence is the existence of a large number of homonyms in the speech of black children that are different from the set of homonyms in the speech system used by the teacher" (Labov, 1970, p. 146).

Black speakers show an extreme degree of *r*-lessness. The /r/ consonant is never found at the end of the word, even though the next word begins with a vowel—while in white New Yorkers or Bostonians the /r/ appears at ends of words if followed by a vowel, e.g. Clara. Thus for blacks, there is no clue for the proper spelling of the /r/ consonant at ends of words, but for whites there is (Labov, 1970, p. 147). There are also some words in which the black speaker will never pronounce the intervocalic /r/ in the middle of the word, thus again having no spelling clues for the /r/ in such words. The /r/ is usually replaced by slight vowel prolongation or a center glide, e.g. Karen becomes "Ka'en." The consonant /l/ is very similar to the /r/ in its phonetic nature, both sounds being liquid. The pattern of /l/ dropping is very similar to that of /r/, and the obscurity of both is more pronounced in black speakers than in white speakers of the same dialectal regions (Labov, 1970, p. 148).

Simplification of consonant clusters is another creolization characteristic of black speech. There is a general tendency to reduce clusters of consonants at the ends of words to a single consonant (Labov, 1970, p. 148). Usually in words ending in /t/ or /d/, the preserved consonant is the first consonant in the cluster, i.e. past becomes "pass," rift becomes "rif," mend becomes "men," etc. When the /l/ is the first member of the cluster, the tendency is to omit it also and the word loses its intelligibility almost completely; for example, wild becomes "wow," and told becomes "toe." In the case of words ending in /s/ or /z/, sometimes the first element of the cluster is preserved and sometimes the second.

Another phonological variation in black speech is the tendency to weaken the final consonants of words. The final /t/ and /d/ are most affected by the tendency. "Final /-d/ may be devoiced to a /t/-like form or disappear entirely. Final /-t/ is often realized as a glottal stop . . . but more often disappears entirely. Less often final /-g/ and /-k/ follow the same route. . . . Final /-m/ and /-n/ usually remain in the form of various degrees of nasalization of the preceding vowel. Rarely, sibilants /-s/ and /-z/ are weakened after vowels" (Labov, 1970, p. 150).

Also black speakers tend to make no distinction between /i/ and /e/ before nasals and liquids, e.g. been often becomes "ben." The final /θ/ is replaced by the /f/ sound and the final /ð/ is replaced by the /v/ sound rather regularly. There are a number of other minor phonological differences, but the aforementioned seem to be the most noticeable variations.

The above phonological variations often involve the same sounds that are reflected in some basic differences in grammatical word inflections. The inflectional variations are not necessarily caused by phonological variations but may be an additional complication. For example, the tendency to omit the /s/ or /z/ in the possessive case is not only found in consonant clusters at the end of words but also after vowels.

The phonological omission of the /l/ sound, however, has a definite effect upon the inflection commonly used for future tenses, i.e. omission of the /l/ in such words as *you'll, they'll,* and *he'll* make them appear to be *you, they,* and *he.* The full form of *will* is used for future, but *going to* is usually replaced by the neutral schwa, as in "I'm a shoot you."

Some additional variations include multiple negation; absence of the copula, especially in the second or third person (such as "he in the way"); no third person singular /s/; no possessive /s/; weak /ed/ suffix; and frequent substitution of the invariant form of *be* for *am, is,* and *are* (such as in "I be tired"). In integrated schools, the phonological variations seem to be overcome more readily by black speakers than the grammatical variations, which seem to remain fairly fixed.

Special note needs to be made that although these patterns are considered typical of the normal linguistic environment of black speakers, they are given special consideration in Chapter 2, when we discuss environmentally different children.

PIDGINIZATION. In the case of the Spanish American and native American speakers whose use of English is mainly as a second language, the English corruptions are considered to be pidginizations since they have not become crystalized as characteristics of the dominant language. However, pidginization seems to have the same devastating influence upon efficiency of social communication and development of reading skills as does creolization in the case of black speakers.

Many Spanish-speaking Americans, for example, especially those in the lower socioeconomic groups, are reported to rarely learn to read past the third and fourth grade level (Peña, 1970, p. 157), though this seems to be less of a problem today than a few years ago. The major characteristics of their spoken English are reduced vocabulary, fragmentation of sentences, and Spanish pronunciation and stress patterns superimposed onto the English constructions. They also tend to adopt some of their own transformational forms rather than those of English, which affects such transformational functions as grammatical word-agreement inflections for number, tense, and person, the genitive form, the auxiliary transformation, and the use of the negative question and passive forms. Mexican American children especially have difficulty with the present tense endings of verbs since "the third person singular is the only tense that ends in /s/" (Hidalgo, 1966, pp. 77-78).

Native American pidginization of English is reflected by reduced vocabulary, fragmentation of sentences, and superimposition of the pronounciation and stress patterns of their own native language upon English patterns. English transformations are also highly influenced by the transformational forms of their own native language—involving important variations in the expression of grammatical word inflections, possessive, auxiliary, negative, question, and passive forms. Some of these latter transformational forms may be more affected than others, such as word-agreement inflections. Since so many different native languages are involved and each has its own peculiar pidginization influence, it is difficult to generalize the differences that exist. Those of the Navajo may serve, however, as illustrative (this is the largest native American linguistic subgroup in the United States).

Indian languages, such as Navajo, share less commonality with English than do French, Spanish, or Italian. Therefore, native Americans seem to have a greater struggle, generally speaking, learning English than Spanish American children (Young, 1970). The phonology of the Navajo language excludes phonemes corresponding to the English /f/, /v/, /θ/, /ð/, and /ŋ/ (Saville, 1970). The English-speaking Navajo child commonly substitutes /b/ for /p/; he often omits the final /d/ or substitutes a glottal stop or the Navajo's version of the /d/. The Navajo /d/ (more like a /t/ than a /d/) is also substituted for /t/ or /d/ in initial positions and for the /ð/ in the middle position. The /ʔ/ is frequently substituted for stop consonants added before initial vowels (Saville, 1970). A gutteral sound is substituted for initial /θ/ and /ð/. The /m/ is substituted for the final /ŋ/ or /n/. English has a greater variety of vowel sounds than Navajo. Navajo does not have the /æ/ and /e/ phonemes, so these are quite difficult for the Navajo child to learn. It is also difficult for the Navajo child to differentiate between /o/, /i/, and /u/ at the appropriate time.

Grammatically, the Navajo child has great difficulty with the stress and pitch contours of English since these are absent or are completely different in the Navajo language. Articles and adjectives are practically nonexistent in the Navajo language. They tend not to differentiate between the English plural and singular form of the noun. The possessive /s/ is also a problem. Third person pronouns are often confused in terms of gender, number, and case.

Many semantic difficulties arise from differences in conceptual classifications. For example, an object or action concept that the

English culture might identify as being the same even when it occurs under varying circumstances may be considered a completely different object or action concept in each differing circumstance in the Navajo culture. *Snow* in the Eskimo culture has numerous labels that represent to them completely different concepts. In the Navajo language, the verb *to give* has at least twelve different forms and the form used depends upon, among other things, the shape of the object involved.

Individual Variations

Earlier we discussed aspects of language shared by all members of the human species that sets it apart as distinctly different from all other animal species. We also discussed aspects of language shared by all members of specific language cultures that set a culture apart as being distinctly different linguistically from all other cultures. In the present section we wish to discuss some aspects of oral language behavior in which each individual differs from each other individual, setting him apart as distinctly different within his own social group. Such differences probably stem from individual differences in biological makeup as well as in the life experiences of the individual. Some of the important ways in which each individual is unique from each other individual are presented briefly below.

Verbal Output: Amount and Quality

"Some people talk a great deal; others speak hardly at all" (Johnson, 1946). This is possibly one of the most obvious ways in which people differ. Verbal output varies in a number of ways. One way in which individuals differ is in the amount of the total waking time that they spend in verbalizing. Since amount of verbal output varies in the same individual from one circumstance to another, categorizing or labeling an individual quantitatively in terms of amount of verbal output is not a very reliable approach unless the person is generally an extremely talkative or extremely quiet individual; in the case of the latter extreme, quantitative assessment is not really necessary since we become readily aware qualitatively of these trait differences in people.

A second way in which individuals vary in verbal output is in terms of vocabulary diversity. Vocabulary diversity can be measured quantitatively by recording a representative portion of a person's verbal output and counting the frequency of occurrence of vocabulary. By dividing the number of different words (types) spoken by the total words (tokens) uttered, a ratio results called the type-token ratio (TTR). Given a certain length of communication on a given topic, a large type-token ratio represents a great deal of diversity. Although the exact relationship between diversity and total size of output vocabulary is not known, it seems logical that degree of diversity would be influenced by size, the greater the size, the more diversity. This logic is somewhat supported by the discrepancy between TTRs of normal and mentally retarded children, the TTR of the latter being lower.

Studies of vocabulary have demonstrated that the more frequently a word is uttered in speech, the shorter it tends to be in terms of number of syllables (Black, 1952). Cherry (1957, p. 180) has suggested that relative frequency of words with varying syllable lengths may be an additional indication of vocabulary diversity. More frequent usage of larger words signals the probability of a greater diversity of vocabulary.

A third type of individual variance in verbal output is in terms of output reflecting intensity and quality of emotional feeling. Gottschalk, Winget, and Gleser (1969) have reported a content analysis of verbal behavior (describing any interesting or dramatic personal life experience) that demonstrates a significant influence of emotion upon the nature of verbal output. Their studies demonstrated that verbal content can be used fairly reliably to differentially identify the presence of abnormal emotional tendencies toward anxiety, hostility, or social alienation (schizophrenia) as follows: (1) verbal content with an unusual preponderance of words or phrases that express or imply fear or guilt concerning one's self suggests an abnormal emotional state of anxiety, (2) verbal content with a preponderance of words or phrases that express or imply destructive, injurious, or critical thoughts and actions directed toward others or toward one's self suggests an abnormal emotional state of hostility, and (3) verbal content with a preponderance of phrases that express or imply an unrealistic, unjustified, or illogical description of the person's relationship with others or with his environmental surroundings suggests an abnormal emotional state of alienation or disorientation. Three subscales designed to measure or assess the above classifications of emotional tendencies have been developed and published (Gottschalk, Winget, and Gleser, 1969). Preliminary studies indicate that the scales have a fairly high reliability value: 0.76 to 0.93 for the anxiety scale, 0.731 to 0.989 for the hostility scale, and 0.94 to 0.90 for the alienation-discrimination scale. If further research substantiates the reliability and validity of this approach to assessment, it should substantiate the fact that verbal output is significantly influenced by the emotional state of the individual and that its degree of emotionality would then vary greatly from one individual to another.

Still another way in which output varies from one individual to another is in terms of intelligibility, i.e. the percentage of what one says that can be interpreted perceptually (with substantial agreement) by a group of listeners who use the same basic language code. Studies have shown that this is a highly individual phenomenon in the so-called average population as well as in deviant groups (Black, 1952; Mecham, 1960).

Semantic and Sequential Memory

Some people can remember numbers, dates, and names almost as if they had a special gift. One of the present authors, on the other hand, has to go through all kinds of torture because of the difficulty he has remembering such things as birthdates, anniversaries, and names of the people he met ten years or so ago while on vacations. Jakobson and Halle (1956) talk about two types of associational cues that are established for symbolic retrieval, i.e. sequential cues and substitutive cues. Given the first type of cuing, in free association the stimulus word *pig* is most likely to be associated with tail or headed due to strong serial bondings of these words in sequence. However if the predominant associational cues are of a substitutive nature, the stimulus word pig will more likely be reacted to in free association through the utterance of a word analogous to pig like hog or sow.

Brown and McNeill (1966) describe a similar dichotomy in memory during efforts to retrieve name words that match with their operational definition. An example was given in which subjects were asked to recall the name of "a navigational instrument used in measuring angle or distances and especially altitude of sun, moon, and stars at sea." The name to be correctly recalled was sextant. The responses of some subjects were apparently cued by substitutive or semantic cues in retrieval since their responses include words with differing sequential patterns but similar meaning, such as astrolobe, compass, dividers, and protractor. Other subjects utilized sequential pattern cues in retrieval and came up with such words as secant, sextet, and sexton.

In a special class demonstration, we presented a short story that was centered around a mystery. The students were subsequently asked to write down the story as completely and accurately as possible. Cursory analysis of the written reports indicated that students who were the most proficient in recalling the correct word or words with similar phonetic patterns to the correct words, left out more of the content of the story than students who recalled content but commonly substituted words similar in meaning but not of the same phonetic pattern as the words used in the story. This suggested that the students were using two different approaches for recall that seem to predominantly utilize either the semantic (analogous) cue approach or the sequential (rote) cue approach.

Miller (1951) has indicated that some people can learn more efficiently through rote memorization (sequential cues) than by content meaning and vice versa—some can learn better by associating the unfamiliar pattern with content meaning (semantic) cues. This ability seems to vary greatly from one individual to another.

Listening Accuracy

Not only does verbal output vary in amount and in accuracy from one individual to another, but verbal input has also recently been determined to be a skill that is highly sensitive to individual differences (Nichols, 1960; Horrworth, 1966; Mecham, 1971).

Nichols described variability of listening skills, at any one grade level, as being as great as variability of reading skills (Nichols, 1957; Nichols and Lewis, 1954). Although the language arts field has traditionally stressed speaking, reading, writing, and spelling as being the important facets of the language arts, in the areas of learning and learning disabilities, recent stress has been placed on the importance of listening.

Zigmond (1969) found dyslexic boys to have more difficulties in auditory perceptual tasks than in visual. Flowers and Crandall (1967) tested five central auditory skills in 287 kindergarten children to see the extent to which these measures could be used as predictors of later academic achievement of the children. The five central auditory skills predicted the children's later academic achievement in reading, general achievement, language, science, social studies, and arithmetic with a high degree of accuracy. Bateman (1969) reported a study on a visual versus an auditory approach to teaching reading to 100 normal children and found the auditory approach to be superior even with children whose strongest modality seemed to be visual. Young (1969) surveyed 700 normal achievers in second, third, fourth, and fifth grades and found that children with the lowest listening accuracy scores differed significantly in reading and academic achievement from children with the highest listening scores. Holloway (1971) matched a group of expressive language delayed children with a group of normal children and found the language delayed group to be different from the control group primarily in auditory perception and in auditory-visual integration. Kirby et al. (1972) found the auditory subtests to be the only ones on the ITPA to be related to reading abilities in a prison population. Golden and Steiner (1969) reported the same thing to be true with second-grade children.

Mecham (1971) demonstrated that listening accuracy is not only a developmental phenomena, i.e. improves systematically in the child with increased age, but it varies considerably from individual to individual and also as a function of the listening situation. He tested 1,800 young elementary-school children in groups of thirty and ninety-six individually using the same listening test procedures. The mean score (M) of second graders (N = 369) in listening for group testing was 72.81 and their standard deviation (SD) was 14.50, while that for individual testing (N = 20) was M = 78.95 and SD = 4.80. Nichols (1960) has outlined a number of factors that he feels are involved in influencing the variability of listening. These included familiarity, values, and interest. Two very important influences that should attract a great deal of research interest are auditory distraction and psychoneurological habituation (tuning out); these two seem to be the most important factors affecting listening variability in many language disordered children.

LANGUAGE DEVELOPMENT IN CHILDREN: EARLY STAGES

There is substantial evidence that language emergence demonstrates a highly predictable maturational or developmental dimension. The fact that milestones of language development have such developmental regularity that they can be chartered on a developmental curve with an incredibly high degree of ordinal consistency among children is highly suggestive that there is a strong biological predisposition for language development in the human species. Lenneberg (1964) has aptly stated that even though we cannot find any historical connection between language families, the onset of speech and language is a very regular phenomena, "appearing at a certain time in the child's physical development and following a fixed sequence of events" (p. 66). Lenneberg views language development as a gradual unfolding of specialized relationships (Lenneberg, 1975).

Normally at the end of the first month of life a human infant produces differentiated vocalizations such as "fussing" or "whining" as a result of wetness or discomfort, rage cries as the result of pain or fear, "coos" and "goos" as an accompaniment of pleasure and satisfaction. At four months, a baby normally produces both vowels and consonants reflexively (Berry, 1969), suggesting that he is getting some control for coordinating breathing, vocalization, and oral-lingual movements. At five to six months, the infant has enough control over his inspiratory/expiratory time ratio (expiration about six times longer than inspiration) to utter strings of nonsense syllables ("babbling"). Vocal play is substantially increased with some recognizable sounds. From six to eight months, self-imitation occupies a large portion of the child's vocal play and intonational patterns resemble more closely those made by the adult. From eight to nine months, the child normally begins to imitate such things as coughing, shaking his head, or waving his hand and reveals increased comprehension by making some correct differential responses (Berry, 1969). Around twelve to fourteen months, the first true words appear. Dale (1972) suggests as criteria for true words: consistent usage, spontaneity, evidence of understanding, and meaningful usage.

By eighteen months of age, a child has normally developed numerous single words and may be attempting word couplets such as "go bye-bye." By his second birthday, he uses short sentences and has a fairly substantial vocabulary (50 to 100 words). Word couplets are not random but adhere to semantic and syntactic rules. Early combinations have been described as consisting usually of two types or classes of words, pivot (P) and open (O) (Braine, 1963). The rules of pivot grammar (Willbrand, 1975) may be written as:

$$ S \rightarrow \left\{ \begin{array}{c} (P_1) + O \\ O + (P_2) \end{array} \right\} $$

Examples of $S \rightarrow P + O$ include word combinations like "see boy," "see sock," and "bye-bye man;" $S \rightarrow O + P_2$ includes combinations like "do it," "shoe off," "move it," etc.

Pivot grammar analysis was used by Braine (1963) to describe the earliest stage of the child's syntactic development. However, this analysis has been thought by some to be inadequate in its description (Bloom, 1970; Slobin, 1971; Brown, 1973). These latter authors have proposed semantic categories as a more adequate description of two word utterances.

Other authors have mentioned the possibility that a pivot grammar analysis may account for an initial stage that appears briefly and is then followed by a stage described by semantic analysis as the two-word utterance stage (Schlesinger, 1971b; Anderson and Willbrand, 1977). Another idea was proposed by Bowerman (1976) who suggested that each child might have individualistic language acquisition strategies, some syntactically oriented and some semantically oriented.

These discussions are theoretical in nature and practical in terms of the most adequate method of analysis; but the researchers are not disagreeing on the phenomenon of regularity of onset or the striking similarity in the process of normal language acquisition for children of various cultures.

Another way of looking at language structure developmentally is in terms of a continually expanding number of sentence elements, with differing numbers representing differing stages of linguistic development (Brown, 1973; Morehead and Ingram, 1973; Crystal, Fletcher, and Garman, 1976)—stage 1 = one-element expressions, stage 2 = two-element expressions, stage 3 = three-element expressions, stage 4 = four-element or more expressions, etc. Brown (1973) feels that lengths of utterances is a good barometer of language development since "everything the child learns about the structure of language has the effect of increasing the length of his sentences" (p. 110).

While the increasing amount of elements in the string of an utterance (from one to four elements) indicates something about language development, we now recognize that further analysis must occur if the language is to be described. For instance, it could be said that a child uses three-element utterances. This same child's three-word utterances might be broken into grammatical sentences composed of a NP + VP such as "I like candy"; modified sentences such as "Daddy go work"; VPs such as "want the baby"; or NPs such as "a good boy." Thus, whether we used the structural description of syntax or the meaning analysis of semantics, modern linguistics has provided a method to describe the language form.

For instance we are now aware that following the two word utterance stage (pivot and/or semantic analysis), the three word utterance stage emerges. This stage consists of separate verb phrases, separate noun phrases, and sentences in both grammatical and modified forms. All of these structures appear at the same time with the verb phrase being dominant (Willbrand and Pinborough, 1977). This has all occurred by about two-and-one-half years of age.

As the child matures the language develops rapidly. Sentences become more complicated. Transformations are used to pose sentences with expanded noun and verb phrases, with various verb tenses, with nouns marked for number, with question inversions, with deletions that allow more efficient sentences, with conjoining links such as *and, or,* and *but* with adjoining links such as *when* and *then,* and with embedding links such as *who* and *that.* A full coverage of the linguistic development of the child is beyond the scope of this book, and indeed of probably any book. However, any person interested in language disorders must first understand the normal linguistic development of children. A few books (Dale, 1976; Menyuk, 1971; Bar-Adon and Leopold, 1971) might provide good starting points. However, most of us are aware that many studies of child language are appearing regularly in journals and as convention papers, and the student of linguistic development needs to keep current by combining for himself the information provided by each study.

While we know that much of language is developed by six years of age, we also know that language acquisition is a continuing process (Willbrand, 1976). Language development continues actively until ten years and certainly beyond although this has not been as clearly defined.

Auditory memory span increases from two to six digits between two-and-a-half and seven years of age; this increase provides a physiological capacity to turn out progressively longer words and longer sentences.

Developmental Issues

Importance of Ordinal Sequencing

Lenneberg (1967) referred to such milestones as those described above as "developmental horizons" representing a whole spectrum of developmental events for which the milestones serve as the most outstanding characteristics. Lenneberg further indicated that if the maturation function is slowed down for some reason, the developmental horizons are reached later and the spacing between milestones is increased without altering the order of their sequence (p. 170). He further noted that differing types of experiences during the course of development do not seem to significantly influence the order of appearance of developmental sequences (p. 9).

The developmental sequencing of perceptual-motor and cognitive milestones in areas outside of the language realm seem to be ordinal, regular, and roughly age dependent, just as language seems to be (Uzgiris and Hunt, 1975). Pure behaviorists, however, are not convinced that ordinal sequence is a critical element in language intervention or development (Guess, Sailor, and Baer, 1974; Gray and Ryan, 1973).

Nature versus Nurture

During the past ten years there has been a strong shift of interest away from the study of formal syntactical structures, such as phrase structure and transformational rules to the study of conditions that form the basis for beginning acquisition of language. Incentive for this shift was possibly facilitated by the unacceptability to many of the theory that language acquisition resulted from the emergence of biologically predetermined (innate) behavior that develops independent of the organisms cognitive abilities (Bowerman, 1976). The nativism proponents (Chomsky, 1965, 1968; Katz, 1966; Lenneberg, 1967; McNeill, 1966, 1970, 1971) suggested that "the child is seen coming to the language learning task equipped with much inborn knowledge of language structure; he requires only a certain amount of linguistic input to activate this knowledge" (Bowerman, 1976, p. 100). Schlesinger (1971a, 1971b) argued, on the other hand, that the basis of early language acquisition results from the child's early efforts to represent his own understandings of the world around him (understandings or concepts that apparently are universal and innate but that are not linguistically dependent and perhaps not even unique to the human species). Ervin-Tripp (1971) suggested that our knowledge of the semantic features characterizing categorical relations "may provide a crucial link in our understanding of how sentences develop" (p. 208). Other searchers have come to strongly support the concept that acquisition of language comes with the discovery of the means by which a child can translate his prelinguistic conceptual notions into words and word combinations (Slobin, 1973; Bloom, 1973; Nelson, 1974; Clark, 1974; Wells, 1974; Miller and Yoder, 1974; Bowerman, 1976).

One of the strong arguments against the nativist point of view that language is not dependent on cognition is that the *"formal structure* of language is not totally distinct from man's more general cognitive organization" (Bowerman, 1976, p. 100). The organization of cognitive structures in general and the organization of language have striking similarities—e.g. categorization, seriation, summation, and embedding. Another argument against the nativist's point of view is that many language categories are dependent upon semantic features that in turn are dependent upon experience and learning (Slobin, 1971).

It is not clear what exact relationships exist between language acquisition and early development of piagetian type, such as object permanence, means strategies, causality, construction, and object interaction (Uzgiris and Hunt, 1975). If relationship categories, such as those suggested by Chafe (1970), Schlesinger (1971a, 1974), Bloom (1970, 1975), etc., are the semantic concepts from which early language emerges, there may be a rather close tie between prelanguage sensorimotor percepts and the emergence of language (Brown, 1973, p. 199). Bloom's (1975) semantic relations categories of *existence, attribute, reoccurrence,* etc., for example, would necessarily require that the child has grasped the concept of object permanence and differentiation. The relational categories of *instrument, intention,* and some form of *action* would assume perceptual knowledge of operational causality and appropriate means of relating to objects and situations.

Assembly versus Differentiation in Development

The more or less traditional differentiation theory, which states that specific behavioral domains of an organism that differ in form and function emerge from a single common generic behavior, has more or less resulted in the assumption that the earliest behaviors to emerge (reflexes and piagetian-type sensorimotor behaviors) must be fairly well developed before other more specific behaviors, such as language, can emerge. However, we have often observed severely physically handicapped children whose reflexes were so abnormal and whose general musculature was so involved as to render the development of normal sensori-motor patterns impossible, and yet who have developed a fairly elaborate language system. In actuality, the assembly theory, which says that various behavioral domains develop as separate entities and converge into more complex behaviors, has more ex-perimental evidence in its favor (Lenneberg, 1967). For exam-ple, stepping movements (hopping reactions) are present long be-fore they can be integrated into ambulation; equilibrium and righting reactions are present as relatively separate and inde-pendent entities for some time before they are needed or can be utilized in balance and protective behaviors; nonsense produc-tions of phonemes become fairly sophisticated in the infant long before these same phonemes are used in production of meaning-ful words.

The idea that various behavioral domains develop rather inde-pendently is fairly well marked by the developmental characteris-tics that seem to be similar across domains; i.e. stages of develop-ment within each domain are ordinally fixed and predictable and the stages seem to be roughly age-locked, the fact that they do de-velop fairly independent is evident in cases where one or another domain is slowed down (e.g. social and language development in autistic children) while the others proceed to develop normally.

Perceptual Deficit Hypothesis

There are those who scoff at the idea of perception forming some kind of basis for language acquisition or disturbance (Rees, 1973; Vellutino et al., 1975). However, a deficit in such processes as decoding information in a sentence one hears is a type of deficit in perception; likewise, the decoding of messages of differing complexity takes a progressively more mature per-ceptual ability on the part of the child. Perceptual and motor processing therefore must be considered important components in the processing of language.

The fallacy in thinking that perhaps led to the objections put forth by Rees and others against the perceptual deficit hypothesis of language disability was the notion on the part of many (Kephart, 1960; Doman et al., 1960; Getman, 1962; Barsch, 1965; Frostig and Maslow, 1973) that the temporal interlocking of language development and the perceptual-motor milestones, or the co-occurrence of perceptual-motor and language disorders, were evidence that the development of such perceptual-motor skills is a prerequisite (and thus a facilitator) to the development of language. There is no proof that this is in any sense true. On the other hand, the decoding and encoding portions of language are perceptual and motor in nature, but the exact nature of how disturbances of these processes affect language must remain speculative until more definite information (on their exact nature) is forthcoming.

Informational Processing Correlates

Lenneberg has suggested that "Language ability should be seen as a process of (a) extracting relations from (or computing relationships in) the physical environment, and (b) of relating these relationships. . . . The thesis . . . is that language knowledge is best represented as a family of processes or, in other words, as cerebral activity states" (Lenneberg, 1975, pp. 17–18).

Models that attempt to explain perceptual and/or motor processing of information in communication have been presented over the past several years (Wathen-Dunn, 1967; Broadbent, 1958; Wepman, 1960; Osgood, 1963; Whitaker, 1971; Sanders, 1976; etc.). Most of these models address themselves to the major components of (1) reception, response of the peripheral sense organ to sensory stimulation pattern; (2) decoding, analysis and identification or restructuring of patterns; (3) interpretation, making decisions regarding appropriate reactions called for, using a conceptual library of experience as the criteria for such decisions; (4) encoding, acting upon one's own conceptual ideas in such a way that they are formed into coded messages designed to convey these ideas to another person or overtly to oneself; and (5) transmission, motor activity that transforms encoded messages into physical patterns that can be picked up by a receiver (thus starting anew the reception part of the cycle).

Although the importance of *attention, rehearsal,* and *memory* in the processing of communication information are mentioned

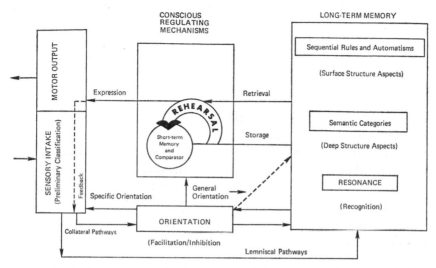

Figure 1. Exploratory model of audiolinguistic processes. From M. J. Mecham and G. A. McCandless, Toward a Model for Analyzing Audiolinguistic Process Dysfunctions in Language Disorders, a paper presented at the 1977 American Speech and Hearing Association Convention, Chicago, Illinois.

by a number of the above model designers, none give an adequate representation of how these processes relate to the total audiolinguistic paradigm. Considerable evidence has been accumulated that suggests that attention, rehearsal, classification, and memory play a primary role in all learning, and therefore must play an important role in language acquisition (Lynn, 1966; Norman, 1969; Morey, 1970; Smythies, 1970; Luria, 1973; Loftus and Loftus, 1976; etc.) and may be seriously affected in language disorders (Berry, 1969; Bannatyne, 1971; Burrows, 1971; Allen, 1971).

Figure 1 is a paradigmatic schema (Mecham and McCandless, 1977) illustrating the interactive roles that attention, rehearsal, classification, and memory play in the processing of audiolinguistic information. These processes are not really steps in language behavior, but may influence each other backward and forward. Any disruption of these basic processing mechanisms may be devastating to the normal development of language.

Pattern Intake and Orientation

When a novel stimulus pattern impinges on the peripheral part of the acoustic analyzer, it normally sets off a series of reflexive arousal and orienting activities in the nervous system. Arousal is an increase in wakefulness, and orientation is an increase in preparedness of the organism for dealing with an external stimulus. These responses are relatively invariant and are affected significantly by the nature of the stimulus pattern.

The initial phase of the attentional response is a generalized reflexive orientation (Lynn, 1966). This is a nonspecific attention involving all modalities. As soon as the significant characteristics of a stimulus pattern are classified (probably within a fraction of a second), there is a funneling or switching of orientation to that specific modality best equipped to handle it. Iconic or visual patterns serve as cues for activation of the visual modality while echoic or auditory patterns cue the activation of the auditory analyzer.

Specific orienting responses on the EEG are strongest to novel or unlearned material and diminish gradually upon repeated exposure of the stimulus; they are strongest at the beginning of the learning (memorizing) cycle and gradually decrease in strength proportional to the strength of learning (Lynn, 1966).

The voluntary component of attention enables us to selectively attend to any of the components of a stimulus that we choose to concentrate on. For example, we can present a figure tachistoscopically that has ten automobiles and ten airplanes and ask a subject to try to determine the number of airplanes within a 0.10 second exposure; if you ask him to tell the number of both the airplanes and automobiles, his estimate of the number of one type of stimulus will be more accurate than his estimate of the number of the other type; which is more accurate will depend upon which stimulus proved to be most interesting. This selectivity of attention may prove to be very important as suggested in our later discussions of disorders of language acquisition.

Attentional vigilance is the attentional monitoring of a stimulus (or stimuli) over a prolonged period of time; the stimulus being monitored may be continuous (as tracking a moving target visually) or discrete (as in noting the number of blocks a stutterer makes in a given period of time).

Auditory voluntary attention can be unilateral (involving only the ear on the right or the left side of the body), bilateral (involving attending to the same stimulus with both ears), or dichotic (listening alternately to the stimulus in one ear and then to a different stimulus in the other ear in order to perceive the stimuli coming in both ears). Most people have a right ear advantage (REA) attentionally—stimuli going in the right ear can more readily be perceived than those going in the left ear.

Recognition (Classification)

Recognition of a stimulus pattern is awareness of the degree to which various elements in the stimulus pattern have been previously conditioned (familiarity). Measured reaction times for recognition have usually averaged around 0.2 second (Sternberg, 1967). It may be that recognition time is much less than that since reaction time involves both recognition and response. Sperling's research (1963) suggests it takes about 0.01 second to recognize the visual pattern of a single letter.

There are a number of reasons for believing that recognition memory is separate from recall memory: (1) Recognition memory is much more efficient than recall memory, i.e. it is much easier to recognize a seldom heard word than to recall it. (2) Recognition is instantaneous (similar to a resonance phenomena as illustrated in Figure 1) and therefore probably does not involve a memory searching process. (3) Maintenance rehearsal (holding information in consciousness) improves recognition memory but does not improve recall memory, while intentional rehearsal (organizing information for future recall) improves recall memory but does not affect recognition memory (Loftus and Loftus, 1976, p. 93). (4) Recall can be affected by retrieval problems while recognition is usually spared (a classic example of this is the amnesic aphasic who cannot recall words voluntarily but can recognize the name of an object without any difficulty; another example is the tip-of-the-tongue phenomenon in which one introspectively cannot recall a word but can recognize immediately whether the listener has guessed the word correctly or incorrectly).

Recognition apparently allows one to cluster the incoming patterns into various "chunks" according to some previously learned or innate frame of reference; this chunking enables one to hold more complex patterns in short-term memory for further processing (Miller, 1956). In this sense, the chunking process in recognition could be considered to be part of the decoding process.

Superficial recognition occurs when elements of a pattern are not very similar to elements in any stored contextual category, while more definitive recognition occurs when a rich identity can be developed between the pattern and the various contexts to which it can relate. If the recognition process tells one that the incoming pattern is novel, or some elements of it are novel, there is an immediate increase or renewal of specific attention arousal.

Short-term Memory

Short-term memory is a momentary (not more than ten seconds) store of the incoming stimulus pattern to enable one to hold it in abeyance until some decision can be made regarding it (maintenance rehearsal) or to organize or recycle it (intentional rehearsal) for storage in long-term memory. Since the recognition process has elicited a match between the incoming stimulus and previously stored experiences, it may be that short-term memory allows time for the conscious regulating mechanisms to perform further processing. Strength of this bonding seems to be a function of the initial strength of the specific orientation response and also of the rate of habituation of that same orienting response.

Short-term memory also allows time for the stimulus pattern to be recycled in the rehearsal process; conversely, material can be held in short-term memory for an indefinite period of time only through the process of rehearsal. (How often have you been given a telephone number and had to look around to find a pencil before writing it down; you find yourself repeating the number over and over to yourself in order not to forget it before you get it written down?) Since rehearsal is the primary process involved in committing sequential or rote aspects of the stimulus pattern to long-term memory, it is quite certain that rehearsal is a functional part of the conscious short-term memory unit.

Imitation is a common (almost invariable) accompaniment of early learning of language. Imitation is made possible through the aid of the recycling process in short-term memory; patterns are maintained long enough in the conscious mechanism for them to be reflected back through the imitative process. Imitation has been recognized in association with language learning longer than any of the processes and yet is probably the least understood of all of the processing mechanisms. More research needs to be directed toward the nature of the role played by imitation in language acquisition (Rees, 1975).

A comparator mechanism in short-term memory (Figure 1) apparently makes it possible for one to monitor his own speech and determine the degree to which his output (actual) patterns matches his input (intended) patterns. This phenomena of self-monitoring strongly suggests that recognition memory occurs early in the processing program, probably prior to as well as during short-term memory processing.

Long-term Memory

There are aspects of long-term memory that are of special importance in communicative behavior: the storage and retrieval of the meaning (deep structure) conveyed by verbal strings—referred to by Tulving (1972) as semantic memory—and the storage of details of the sequential structure of the pattern (surface structure).

By use of semantic memory, we are able to retell the most meaningful parts of a long story after we have heard it only once, although the words we use are likely to be radically different from the words that we heard. In fact, to retell a story in the exact same words requires considerably more repetition than a single hearing—the more exacting the match, the greater the number of repetitions required, as a rule.

Semantic memory seems to react to cues that activate memories of past experiences categorically. Once the categorical memory or concept has been activated, the original cues (whether visual or auditory) can be discarded or forgotten without forgetting the concept.

Memory for exact verbal-string structure, however, has a greater dependency upon the raw material being transferred from the sensory intake component than it does upon the experiential or conceptual store and therefore requires a much greater amount of repetition or rehearsal for its precise storage. This latter type of processing, as mentioned earlier, is highly dependent upon the functions of the mechanisms of the short-term memory component.

Storage and retrieval in long-term memory are two important processes in communicative behavior that we do not fully understand. However, difficulties in storing and/or retrieving may be central to the processing problems of language disordered children. In fact, many language disordered children seem to have a major difficulty in temporally processing rapidly occurring acoustic events (Tallal, Stark, and Curtiss, 1976). Whether this is a disorder of intake selectivity and sensory store, short-term memory store, recognition reaction time, or some other processing mechanism is not clear.

Motor Output

We know very little about the encoding process in language, although a great deal is known about its final common pathway—speech. We know that language is the precursor to speech and that it culminates in the so-called surface structure, that, in the case of spoken language, is finally propagated phonetically. The first phase of the encoding process in language is the formation of an idea or thought that needs to be expressed (MacNeilage and Ladefoged, 1976). The second phase is arranging the idea or thought in terms of appropriate representational symbols; in verbal language, this has to be a phrase or a sentence comprised of appropriate lexical items, arranged in proper semantic and syntactic sequence and utilizing the proper phonological rules.

The third phase of the language-speech encoding chain is the organization of a plan or neuromotor coordinations (praxis) that will produce the phonetic and phonological patterns necessary to convey the linguistic code. The fourth phase is the execution of the actual motor patterns ordered by this plan. The physiological and mechanical processes used in this fourth phase (speech production) have received considerable attention in terms of both normal and disordered function (Darley, Aronson, and Brown, 1975; MacNeilage and Ladefoged, 1976; Hardcastle, 1976).

Introspectively, the first phase (ideation) and the fourth phase (final motor production) are the phases of which the speaker and the listener seem most consciously aware; and both of these phases have traditionally received the greatest amount of scholarly attention in the fields of education and speech pathology. Much less progress has been made in the second (linguistic programming) and the third (motor programming) phases of encoding.

Liberman (1973) has argued rather convincingly that representation for encoding (and decoding) syllables is in the form of a specialized physiological device that functions in a unique way in humans and specifically for speech; such a device is probably located mainly in the left hemisphere and its function for decoding is perhaps reciprocally analogous to its function in encoding. Liberman accordingly argues that in the production of a word, we do not formulate the beginning, intermediate, and final segments "in tandem, first one and then the other," but, rather, we begin the formulation of all of the segments at about the same time. No other animal is capable of this complex but efficient coordination; yet it is so easy for human beings "that one-year-old infants do it quite expertly in their spontaneous babbling" (p. 134). According to Liberman, the resulting sound of an articulated word is different from the sound formed in any other way, i.e. it is "at every instant, transmitting information simultaneously about more than one segment of the phonetic message" (p. 135). No other type of acoustic message, e.g. Morse code, can be perceived and analyzed as rapidly as the acoustic message that has been spoken. "There is now a great deal of evidence that we as human beings do, in fact, possess a special speech decoder. We don't know yet exactly how this decoder works, but we know what it has to do" (p. 135). Liberman's postulation about humans having a specialized decoder is strengthened by studies in dichotic listening that show that there is a right ear advantage in man for speech only. It also suggests a possibility of a counterpart in the form of a special speech encoder that makes possible the incredibly complex and rapidly occurring neuromuscular coordinations involved in speech.

SUMMARY

This chapter has presented rather detailed descriptions of a child's linguistic foundations, which are comprised of universal, culture-specific, subcultural, and individual variations. It also discusses briefly the early stages of language development in children, developmental issues, and informational processing correlates to the learning of language. The next chapter describes some of the major disorders of language in children.

References

Allen, J.: The effects of covert and overt rehearsal on children's imitation of meaningful and nonmeaningful speech. Unpublished master's thesis, University of Utah, Salt Lake City, 1971.

Anderson, R. L. and Willbrand, M. L.: Pivot grammar: A forgotten minority. Paper presented at the American Speech and Hearing Association annual convention, Chicago, Illinois, November 1977.

Bannatyne, A.: *Language, reading, and learning disabilities.* Springfield: Thomas, 1971.

Bar-Adon, A. and Leopold, W. F. (Eds.): *Child language: A book of readings.* Englewood Cliffs, New Jersey: P-H, 1971.

Barsch, R. H.: *A movigenic curriculum.* State Department of Public Instruction, publication no. 25, Madison, Wisconsin, 1965.

Bateman, B.: Reading: A controversial view. In Tornopol, L. (Ed.): *Learning disabilities.* Springfield: Thomas, 1969.

Berry, M. F.: *Language disorders of children.* New York: Appleton-Century-Crofts, 1969.

Black, J. W.: Accompaniments of word intelligibility. *J Speech Hear Disord, 17:*409-418, 1952.

Bloom, L.: *Language development: Form and function in emerging grammars.* Cambridge, Massachusetts: MIT Pr, 1970.

Bloom, L.: *One word at a time: The use of single-word utterances before syntax.* Cambridge, Massachusetts: MIT Pr, 1973.

Bloom, L.: Structure and variation in child language. *Monogr Soc Res Child Dev, 40*(Serial No. 160): 2, 1975.

Bowerman, M.: Semantic factors in the acquisition of rules for word use and sentence construction. In Morehead, D. M. and Morehead, A. E. (Eds.): *Normal and deficient child language.* Baltimore: University Park, 1976.

Braine, M. D. S.: The ontogeny of English phrase structure: The first phrase. *Language, 39:*1-13, 1963.

Broadbent, D. E.: *Perception and communication.* New York: Pergamon, 1958.

Brown, R.: *A first language: The early stages.* Cambridge, Massachusetts: Harvard U Pr, 1973.

Brown, R. and McNeill, D.: The "tip of the tongue" phenomenon. *J Verbal Learning and Verbal Behavior, 5*:325-337, 1966.

Burrows, C. L.: A comparison of attentional vigilance performance between normal and language delayed subjects. Unpublished master's thesis, University of Utah, Salt Lake City, 1971.

Cazden, C. B.: The psychology of language. In Travis, L. E. (Ed.): *Handbook of speech pathology and audiology.* New York: Appleton-Century-Crofts, 1971.

Chafe, W. L.: *Meaning and the structure of language.* Chicago: U of Chicago Pr, 1970.

Cherry, C.: *On human communication.* New York: McGraw, 1957.

Chomsky, N.: *Syntactic structures.* Hague: Mouton, 1957.

Chomsky, N.: *Aspects of the theory of syntax.* Cambridge, Massachusetts: MIT Pr, 1965.

Chomsky, N.: *Language and mind.* New York: Harcourt, Brace, & World, 1968.

Chomsky, N. and Halle, M.: *The sound patterns of English.* New York, Har-Row, 1968.

Clark, E.: Some aspects of the conceptual basis for first language acquisition. In Schiefelbusch, R. L. and Lloyd, L. L. (Eds.): *Language perspectives: Acquisition, retardation, and intervention.* Baltimore, Maryland: Univ Park, 1974.

Crystal, D., Fletcher, P., and Garman, M.: *The grammatical analysis of language disability.* New York: Elsevier, 1976.

Dale, P. S.: *Language development: Structure and function.* Hinsdale, Illinois: Dryden Pr, 1972.

Dale, P. S.: *Language development: Structure and function* (2nd ed.). Hinsdale, Illinois: Dryden Pr, 1976.

Darley, F. L., Aronson, A. E. and Brown, J. R.: *Motor speech disorders.* Philadelphia: Saunders, 1975.

Doman, R., Spitz, E., Zucman, E., Delacato, C., and Doman, G.: Children with severe brain injuries: Neurological organization in terms of mobility. *JAMA, 174*:257-262, 1960.

Ervin-Tripp, S.: An overview of theories of grammatical development. In Slobin, D. L. (Ed.): *The ontogenesis of grammar.* New York: Acad Pr, 1971.

Flowers, A. and Crandall, E. W.: Relations among central auditory abilities, socioeconomic factors, speech delay, phonic abilities and reading achievement: A longitudinal study. Office of Education Cooperative Research Project, no. 6-8313 (unpublished), Grand Blanc, Michigan, 1967.

Frostig, M. and Maslow, P.: *Learning problems in the classroom.* New York: Grune, 1973.

Getman, G. N.: *How to develop your child's intelligence.* Luverne, Minnesota: Getman, 1962.

Gleason, H. A., Jr.: *An introduction to descriptive linguistics.* New York: HR&W, 1961.

Golden, N. and Steiner, S.: Auditory and visual functions in good and poor readers. *J Learning Disabilities, 2:*476-481, 1969.

Gottschalk, L. A., Winget, C. N., and Gleser, G. C.: *Manual of instructions for using the Gottschalk-Gleser analysis scales.* Berkeley: U of Cal Pr, 1969.

Gray, B. and Ryan, B.: *A language program for the nonlanguage child* Champaign, Illinois: Res Pr, 1973.

Guess, D., Sailor, W. and Baer, D. M.: To teach language to retarded children. In Schiefelbusch, R. L. and Lloyd, L. L. (Eds.): *Language perspectives: Acquisition, retardation, and intervention.* Baltimore, Maryland: Univ Park, 1974.

Hardcastle, W. J.: *Physiology of speech production.* New York: Acad Pr, 1976.

Hidalgo, F.: A reading program for Mexican-American children. HEW first interim report, project no. 5-0559, contract no. OE-6-85-070, Washington, D.C.: US Govt Ptg, 1966.

Holloway, G. E.: Auditory-visual integration in language-delayed children. *J Learning Disabilities, 4:*204-208, 1971.

Horrworth, G. L.: Listening: A facet of oral language. *Elementary English Review, 868:*856-864, 1966.

Hunt, M.: Implications of sequential order in hierarchy in early psychological development. In Friedlander, B. Z., Sterritt, G. M. and Kirk, G. E. (Eds): *Exceptional infant,* vol. 31, *Assessment and intervention.* New York: Brunner-Mazel, 1975.

Jacobs, R. A. and Rosenbaum, P. S.: *English transformational grammar.* Waltham, Massachusetts: Blaisdell, 1968.

Jakobson, R. and Halle, M.: *Fundamentals of language.* Hague: Mouton, 1956.

Johnson, W.: *People in quandaries.* New York: Harper and Brothers, 1946.

Katz, J. T.: *The philosophy of language.* New York: Har-Row, 1966.

Kephart, N.: *The slow learner in the classroom.* Columbus, Ohio: Merrill, 1960.

Kessler, C.: *The acquisition of syntax in bilingual children.* Washington, D.C.: Georgetown U Pr, 1971.

Kirby, E. A., Lyle, W., and Amble, B. R.: Reading and psycholinguistic processes of inmate problem readers. *J Learning Disabilities, 5:*295-298, 1972.

Labov, W.: Language characteristics of blacks. In Horn, T. D. (Ed.): *Reading for the disadvantaged.* New York: HarBrace J, 1970.

Lenneberg, E. H.: *New directions in the study of language.* Cambridge, Massachusetts: MIT Pr, 1964.

Lenneberg, E. H.: *Biological foundations of language.* New York: Wiley, 1967.

Lenneberg, E. H.: The concept of language differentiation. In Lenneberg, E. H. and Lenneberg, E. (Eds.): *Foundations of language development.* New York: Acad Pr, 1975.

Liberman, A. M.: The speech code. In Miller, G. A. (Ed.): *Communication, language, and meaning.* New York Basic, 1973.

Loftus, G. R. and Loftus, E. F.: *Human memory: The processing of information.* New York: Wiley, 1976.

Luria, A. R.: *The working brain.* New York: Basic, 1973.

Lynn, R.: *Attention, arousal, and the orientation reaction.* New York: Pergamon, 1966.

MacNeilage, P. and Ladefoged, P.: The production of speech and language. In Carterette, E. E. and Friedman, M. P. (Eds.): *Handbook of perception,* vol. 7, *Language and speech.* New York: Acad Pr, 1976.

McNeill, D.: Developmental psycholinguistics. In Smith, F. and Miller, G. (Eds.): *The genesis of language.* Cambridge, Massachusetts: MIT Pr, 1966.

McNeill, D.: *The acquisition of language.* New York: Har-Row, 1970.

McNeill, D.: The capacity for grammatical development in children. In Slobin, D. I. (Ed.): *The ontogenesis of grammar: Some facts and several theories.* New York: Acad Pr, 1971.

Mecham, M. J. (Ed.): *Speech therapy in cerebral palsy.* Springfield: Thomas, 1960.

Mecham, M. J.: Measurement of verbal listening accuracy in children. *Learning Disabilities, 4:*257-259, 1971.

Mecham, M. J. and McCandless, G. A.: Toward a modal for analyzing audiolinguistic process dysfunctions in language disorders. Paper delivered at the American Speech and Hearing Association annual convention, Chicago, Illinois, November 1977.

Menyuk, P.: *The acquisition and development of language.* Englewood-Cliffs, New Jersey: P-H, 1971.

Miller, G. A.: *Language and communication.* New York: McGraw, 1951.

Miller, G. A.: The magical number seven, plus or minus two: Some limits on our capacity to process information. *Psychol Rev, 63:*81-97, 1956.

Miller, J. F. and Yoder, D. E.: An ontogenetic language teaching strategy for retarded children. In Schiefelbusch, R. L. and Lloyd, L. L. (Eds.): *Language perspectives: Acquisition, retardation, and intervention.* Baltimore, Maryland: Univ Park, 1974.

Moray, N.: *Attention: Selective processes in vision and hearing.* New York: Acad Pr, 1970.

Morehead, D. M. and Ingram, D.: The development of base syntax in normal and linguistically deviant children. *J Speech Hear Res, 16:*330-352, 1973.

Nelson, K.: Concept, word, and sentence: Interrelations in acquisition and development. *Psychol Rev, 81:*267-285, 1974.

Nichols, R.: What can be done about listening? *Supervisor's notebook*. New York: Scott F, service bulletin 22:1-4, 1960.

Nichols, R. G. and Lewis, T. R.: *Listening and speaking: A guide to effective oral communication*. Dubuque, Iowa: Wm C. Brown, 1954.

Nichols, R. G. and Stevens, L. A.: *Are you listening?* New York: McGraw, 1957.

Norman, D. A.: *Memory and attention: An introduction to human information processing*. New York: Wiley, 1969.

Osgood, C. E. and Miron, M. S. (Eds.): *Approaches to the study of aphasia*. Urbana, Illinois: U of Ill Pr, 1963.

Peña, A. A.: Language characteristics of Spanish speakers. In Horn, T. D. (Ed.): *Reading for the disadvantaged*. New York: HarBrace J, 1970.

Rees, N. S.: Auditory processing factors in language disorders: A view from Procrustes' bed. *J Speech Hear Disord, 38*:305-315, 1973.

Rees, N. S.: Imitation and language development: Issues and clinical implications. *J Speech Hear Disord, 40*:339-350, 1975.

Riessman, G.: *The culturally deprived child*. New York: Har-Row, 1962.

Sanders, D. A.: A model of communication. In Lloyd, L. L. (Ed.): *Communication assessment and intervention strategies*. Baltimore, Maryland: Univ Park, 1976.

Saville, M. R.: Language and the disadvantaged. In Horn, T. D. (Ed.): *Reading for the disadvantaged*. New York: HarBrace J, 1970.

Schlesinger, I. M.: Learning grammar: From pivot to realization rule. In Huxley, R. and Ingram, E. (Eds.): *Language acquisition Models and methods*. New York: Acad Pr, 1971a.

Schlesinger, I. M.: Production of utterances and language acquisition. In Slobin, D. I. (Ed.): *The ontogenesis of grammar*. New York: Acad Pr, 1971b.

Schlesinger, I. M.: Relational concepts underlying language. In Schiefelbusch, R. L. and Lloyd, L. L. (Eds.): *Language perspectives: Acquisition, retardation, and intervention*. Baltimore, Maryland: Univ Park, 1974.

Slobin, D. I.: *Psycholinguistics*. Glenview, Illinois: Scott F, 1971.

Slobin, D. I.: Cognitive prerequisites for the development of grammar. In Ferguson, C. A. and Slobin, D. I. (Eds.): *Studies of child language development*. New York: HR&W, 1973.

Smythies, J. R.: *Brain mechanisms and behavior*. New York: Acad Pr, 1970.

Sperling, G.: A model for visual memory tasks. *Hum Factors, 5*:19-39, 1963.

Sternberg, S.: Memory-scanning: Mental processes revealed by reaction-time experiments. *Am Sci, 57*:421-457, 1967.

Tallal, P., Stark, R. E., and Curtiss, B.: Relation between speech perception and speech production impairment in children with developmental dysphasia. *Brain and Language, 3*:305-317, 1976.

Taylor, O. L.: Some sociolinguistic concepts of black language. *Today's Speech, 19*:19-26, 1971.

Tulving, E.: Episodic and semantic memory. In Tulving, E. and Donaldson, W. (Eds.): *Organization of memory.* New York: Acad Pr, 1972.

Uzgiris, I. C. and Hunt, M.: *Assessment in infancy: Ordinal scales of psychological development.* Urbana, Illinois: U of Ill Pr, 1975.

Vellutino, F. R., Steger, B. M., Moyer, S. C., Harding, C. J., and Niles, J. A.: Has the perceptual deficit hypothesis led us astray? *Journal of Learning Disabilities, 10:*375-385, 1975.

Wathen-Dunn, W. (Ed.): *Models for the perception of speech and visual form.* Cambridge, Massachusetts: MIT Pr, 1967.

Well, G.: Learning to code experience through language. *J Child Language, 1:*243-269, 1974.

Wepman, J. J., Beck, R. D., and Van Polt, D.: Studies in aphasia: Background and theoretical formulations. *J Speech Hear Disord, 25:*468-477, 1960.

Whitaker, H.: Neurolinguistics. In Dingwall, W. O. (Ed.): *A survey of linguistic science.* College Park, Maryland: U of Md Pr, 1971.

Willbrand, M. L.: The case for establishing pivot grammar. In Sharifi, H. (Ed.): *From Meaning to Sound.* Lincoln, Nebraska: U of Nebr Pr, 1975.

Willbrand, M. L.: Language acquisition: the continuing development from nine to ten years. In Ingemann, F. (Ed.): *Mid-America Linguistics Conference Papers.* Lawrence, Kansas: U of Kan, 1976.

Willbrand, M. L. and Pinborough, J.: The prominence of the verb in child language. In Brown, R., Houlihan, K., Hutchinson, L., and MacLeish, A. (Eds.): *Proceedings of the 1976 mid-America linguistics conference.* Minneapolis, Minnesota: U of Minn, 1977.

Young, A. O.: A study of a measure of listening accuracy and reading. Unpublished master's thesis, University of Utah, Salt Lake City, 1969.

Young, R. W.: Language characteristics of American Indians. In Horn, T. D., (Ed.): *Reading for the disadvantaged.* New York: HarBrace J, 1970.

Zigmond, N. K.: Auditory processes in children. In Tarnopol, L. (Ed.): *Learning disabilities.* Springfield, Thomas, 1969.

Chapter 2

LANGUAGE DISORDERS

S PEECH CLINICIANS need to know how to diagnose and treat the
various disorders of oral communication. The child in the
clinical setting will exhibit oral performance that deviates from
the normal children in such a manner that it interferes with communication and/or calls attention to itself. We have traditionally
tended to describe our clients as having articulatory disorders,
voice disorders, fluency disorders, language disorders, etc. If the
use of the term disorders means "a lack of order or regular ar-
rangement; a confusion" (Morris, 1969), then this label may be
inappropriate for most children with language disorders. Increasing evidence has been presented indicating that the language
problems of many children represent patterns that are similar to
child language in normal children of a younger age (Morehead
and Morehead, 1976). In other words, these problems tend to be
represented more by delay than by deviance. Other children present problems of language differences that may be problems to
be treated but do not necessarily represent either delay or deviance. Some children, however, do demonstrate unusual, deviant
patterns of language performance. We can encompass all of
these children if we interpret the term disorder to mean "an upset of health or functioning" (Morris, 1969).

The global area of language disorder then will include all children with language problems. It could be argued that it is more
satisfactory to say that a child has a language problem. The term
language problem may be a more encompassing label that presents the difficulty in a clearer manner than the disorder label. In
addition, as speech pathologists we are concerned with oral language including reception, comprehension, and production. However, we are not, by and large, trained to diagnose or treat language problems involving reading or writing. Thus, we might
most accurately say that a child we are seeing has an oral language problem or disorder.

Our main concern is to avoid any of the old worn-out labels that have no meaning, that need to be explained, or that may be open to an inaccurate interpretation. For some reason, in the area of child language we began using more specific and confusing terminology. For instance, a few years ago under type of problem, we saw labels such as "aphasic" or "autistic." These were examples of etiological terminology. To say someone is aphasic or autistic did not describe the language behavior of that person and did little to guide language treatment. In fact, the use of these terms for the disorders of children may or may not have defined the etiology. Consequently, what followed was years of arguments about labels—arguments typified by those at Stanford in 1960 (West, 1962)—and the clinician was forced to spend time trying to justify the label. Then we little bettered our situation by trying labels like "delayed" or "deviant," which also had to be explained.

To say a child has deviant language, the clinician must prove how the language of this child is deviant as opposed to delayed. Then, if the child also has some signs of delay, the clinician must explain this as an additional problem. The use of the general term language disorder or language problem instead of terms such as delayed language or deviant language enables the clinician to globally define a problem in a term that will be recognized as a broad term. The obvious analogy to this is to say the child has an articulation problem.

When a child has an articulatory problem, we would probably laugh to see a speech clinician writing in a diagnostic report that a child had a problem of "baby talk," "lalling," or "oral inaccuracy" instead of saying the child had an articulatory disorder. Of course, after the clinician stated the general articulatory disorder, he would then define the disorder by stating that the child is substituting /t/ for /k/, /d/ for /g/, /θ/ for /s/, etc.

At this time we are proposing a similar solution in the language area. The clinician would state that a certain child had a language disorder, then the disorder could be described in terms of the details of the pragmatic, semantic, syntactic, and phonologic problems. After the language problem is specified, the clinician would be able to augment the information with a description of any accompanying symptom, such as various physical and behavioral signs.

However, unlike articulation problems, the diagnosis of language disorders is not based on deviation from a set of norms. The reason is simple. There are no adequate norms available in language acquisition. Norms are available for children's performances on certain language tests (see Chapter 3 for discussion) just as norms are available for articulation tests. While a developmental language sequence is predictable, there are no chronological age norms available for specific language forms; that is, there are no tables were we see X structure acquired by X age. Several reasons exist for this problem. The study of children's acquisition of language based on the new methods of language analysis is in its infancy. Most of the research data up to this time consists of studies of a small number of children (sometimes one child is the only subject), usually from higher or middle socioeconomic level families. Additionally, language development is most frequently described by stages rather than by specific structures or categories. All the syntactic structures and semantic categories and any method of describing children's acquisition of language have not been defined any more than such breakdowns have been defined by linguists for grammars. Speech clinicians, therefore, cannot approach the study of language disorders expecting a discussion of how far one must deviate from the norm of a specified developmental sequence. The task of specifying a language problem must be preceded by an understanding and continuous reading of studies on normal language development. Soon a broad sequence begins to emerge—a few authors have summarized these sequences in script (P. Dale, 1976), in tables (Hannah, 1974), and in profile charts (Crystal, Fletcher, and Garman, 1976). However, the clinician should be cautioned against assuming any listings are absolute or normative.

Even with these problems in mind, the certainty is that knowledge of normal language development and of language disabilities is rapidly increasing and is far ahead of where the field was a few years ago. It seems possible to present a description of language problems insofar as current knowledge allows us to proceed. In this chapter on language disorders, the various language problems of children that contribute to a language disorder are discussed. Then the types of children who have language problems are discussed.

LANGUAGE PROBLEMS

The language problems of children are a multifaceted phenomena. The different categories of language problems may exist in varying degrees across all groups of children. The types of language problems are cognitive, semantic, syntactic, phonologic, and pragmatic. Any dichotomy of the components of language or of language problems is, of course, artificial. These problems are separated for clarity of discussion. The language disorder of a given child could be exemplified by problems in any of the following areas in various combinations of areas, or in all of them.

Cognitive Problems

Cognition refers to the mental abilities that enable a person to be aware, to conceptualize, to associate, to understand and, thus, to know. Cromer (1976, p. 289) referred to cognition as bipartate with cognition referring to "thoughts, intentions, and meanings" and cognitive structures as the "underpinning of these thoughts." The interrelationship between language and thought has been the source of philosophical arguments for decades (see Piaget, 1952 and Vygotsky, 1962). Deciding which comes first, language or thought, resembles the chicken and the egg argument. The best solution seems to be to consider the reciprocal relationship of cognition and language. From this perspective, a cognitive problem will surely be, at least in part, manifested as a language problem. Slobin (1973) has developed a detailed postulation about how cognitive development affects both the "meanings" and the "forms" of children's utterances.

Cognitive problems may be represented in various patterns. The child may have difficulties relating to his environment. Difficulties in conceptualizing and abstracting are usually discussed. Problems represented by reduced memory capacity (long-term and short-term) and difficulty with sequencing and temporal order are considered. A more detailed discussion of the involvement of these cognitive processes in central nervous system impaired children is presented later in this chapter.

A basic cognitive underpinning of language seems to be the ability to categorize. Lenneberg (1967) has said that language is a process of categorization. Cognitive misrepresentations of the world, inability to denote distinguishing characteristics, memory problems, and lack of ability to abstract are naturally going to affect one's ability to categorize.

Discussions of the cognitive problems of children are widely available and will range from discussions of overall reduction of abilities, such as appear in mentally retarded children, to discussions of lesser general problems, to discussions of specific disabilities that combine to represent a pattern.

Semantic Problems

The semantic component of language interprets the meaning of a word, a phrase, a sentence, a group of sentences, or a message. Individual interpretation of meaning may reflect the way that person perceives the reality of the world. Thus, in the process of human communication we should expect some normal variation in the conception of meaning. Children with problems in semantics will have disorders in the interpretation of meaning that are outside the bounds of normal.

Semantic disorders remain almost an abstraction at this time. Most conclusions about children's language should be considered exploratory at this time, and the research in semantic development is especially tenuous. Bowerman (1976) recently pointed out that the results of studies on semantic classifications have conflicted. The problem seems to be confounded by the variety of and differences among various methods of semantic categorization as well as by the fact that some children may be using a method of categorization that does not fit any preconceived method of division. Bowerman concluded that only further research would indicate whether semantic concepts actually do play a role in child language acquisition or whether semantic categories are a "convenient vocabulary" for the researcher (p. 155).

In the study of normal development, Bloom (1970), R. Brown (1973), Schlesinger (1971), and Slobin (1971) have presented tables of semantic categories primarily to account for the two-word stage that represented the data they had available. Although the semantic classifications vary somewhat, the concept remains the same—that children's utterances can be classified by meaning relations. The variety in classification systems may be demonstrated by two examples. Slobin (1971, pp. 44-45) used the following categories with these samples from English:

Locate, name	"there book"
Demand, desire	"more milk"
Negate	"no wet"
Describe event or situation	"Bambi go"
Indicate possession	"my shoe"
Modify, qualify	"pretty dress"
Question	"where ball"

Schlesinger (1971, pp. 73-78) proposed position rules with the following examples:

Agent + action	"Bambi go"
Action + direct object	"see sock"
Agent + direct object	"Eve lunch" (Eve is having lunch)
Modifier + head	"pretty boat"
Negation + X	"no wash"
X + dative	"throw daddy" (throw it to daddy)
Introducer + X	"it ball"
X + location	"baby highchair" (baby is in the highchair)

Speech pathologists have begun to report diagnostic and clinician tools utilizing some of the previously mentioned classification systems (MacDonald and Blott, 1974; Miller and Yoder, 1974) appearing concurrently with the classifications for semantic disorders. These methods have been presented with the assumption that children do have semantic problems. However, Freedman and Carpenter (1976) using these same classification systems (basically Schlesinger's) reported that when language impaired children were matched with normal children for stage of language acquisition "the language impaired group expressed the same semantic relations with as much variability and flexibility as the normal group" (p. 792).

In considering semantic problems of older children, the information is equally confusing. Chappell (1972) discussed certain aspects of language problems. While he did not specifically label his categories as semantic disorders, a few of the characteristics seem to specify semantic problems. For instance, the child may be aware of one meaning of a word but not of all the variety of meanings. As an example, he mentions expressions using the word *fair* with various meanings, such as "the local fall animal fair," "My, doesn't Mary have fair hair," and "It looks like it is going to be a fair day." Chappell also mentions problems in expressing similarities and differences as well as word association, word classifying, and cause and effect relationships. He said that all of these differences are subtle and difficult to catch, but often result in problems in communication.

However, Willbrand (1976) reported that normal children from nine to ten years of age were also demonstrating problems in message communication. These children used sentences that demonstrated limited semantic interpretation of a word. For instance, most of the subjects interpreted *beyond* in terms of distance and did not consider the definition of time. Thus, the sentence "You go to college beyond high school" was interpreted as distance, and the sentence "I can get the ball back three out of four times" was usually interpreted to mean one time because the children substracted three from four to understand the sentence. The normal children were also using unique interpretations as in "my voice is horny" (defined as hoarse), coined words, and combining new words. Speech pathologists should beware of assuming an older child has disordered language when he demonstrates limited or unique meaning interpretation.

Describing semantic problems at this time seems a difficult chore, but one that we are trying to surmount. Any method used at this time should probably be considered experimental. (For a more complete discussion of the problems of semantic categories see Bowerman, 1976; Miller and McNeill, 1969; and Willbrand, 1977b.) All the confusion, however, should not necessarily preclude the clinician's awareness of the possibility of semantic problems.

Syntactic Problems

The syntactic component of language is concerned with the finite set of rules specifying how elements may be strung together to make sentences. Linguists are offering a variety of grammars (such as generative or case) to describe that finite set of rules that is the basis for an infinite number of human utterances.

Since the late 1950s, the work of linguists has been predicated (either in acceptance or refutation) on the theories of Noam Chomsky (1957, 1965). The theoretical issues as well as data based studies of child language have been concerned with the importance of syntax to human language. Whether or not linguistic theorists have agreed to the Chomskian suggestion of the centrality of syntax to human language, the crucial importance of syntax has been recognized. Yet as linguistic theorists and those involved in study of child language have been struggling to describe language syntactically, those working in language disorders have not been as specific in describing the language problems of children.

Crystal, Fletcher, and Garman (1976) said, "Syntax has come to be seen as the network of organization principles underlying linguistic expression, without which language would become an incoherent jumble of vocabulary and sound. It would accordingly be surprising if language disorders did not need to be related to syntax in some fundamental way; and it is surprising when one discovers how little attention has in fact been focused on this point" (p. 5).

The lack of attention to syntactic disorders may stem from speech clinicians waiting for linguists to decide that one grammar is the answer or for developmental norms in syntax to be established. As it becomes apparent that both of these are unrealistic expectations, more studies on descriptions and treatments of syntactic disorders seem likely.

Certainly, more is known about normal children's acquisition of syntax than any other component of language. Since the emergence of Chomsky, the study of syntax has received and continues to receive a great deal of attention. Studies of normal children's acquisition as well as syntactic theories have been in abundance since 1957, while studies on language disorders have remained scarce.

Some of the initial efforts to describe syntactic disorders concentrated on whether the children with disorders demonstrated deviant development, and these reports presented conflicting conclusions. For instance, Lenneberg, Nichols, and Rosenberger (1964) and Lackner (1968) reported that children with language problems demonstrated syntactic development similar to normal children, while Menyuk (1964) and Lee (1966) concluded that disordered children used structures that were dissimilar from normally developing children. After these initial efforts, it became apparent to researchers that these children were being compared by chronological ages rather than by language age. More recent researchers have compared the syntactic patterns of normal and disordered children representing the same language age, disregarding the chronological age. The study by Morehead and Ingram (1973) is representative of studies matching children by stage of syntactic development and they concluded, "Linguistically deviant children do not develop bizarre linguistic systems that are qualitatively different from normal children. Rather, they develop quite similar linguistic systems with a marked delay in the onset and acquisition time. Moreover, once the linguistic systems are developed, deviant children do not use them as creatively as normal children for producing highly varied utterances" (p. 344).

At the current time we might conclude that most children with syntactic problems will demonstrate structural language that is like that of a younger child but does not contain as many novel or creative utterances. However, the problem is more complicated than this.

Crystal, Fletcher, and Garman (1976, pp. 113-117) presented "patterns of syntactic disorders." This grouping seemed to express differences in children with language disorders that have not been explicit in the research.

Pattern one was the delayed language profile. In this group, the language of the child was well balanced in structure but was typical of a younger child. They felt this pattern was usually found in educational settings where children were from "disadvantaged" homes. More specifically, the child with pattern one would present a language profile like a normal younger child. The child would be talking enough and have a distribution of utterances presenting a variety of normal structures. Thus a four-and-a-half-year-old child might demonstrate a few single-word utterances composed of nouns or verbs; two-word utterances composed of subject + verb, verb + object, noun + noun, verb + verb, or verb + participle; three-element utterances consisting of subject + verb + object, verb + complement, and subject + verb + adverbial, as well as determiner + adjective + noun. This child would also demonstrate four-element or more sentences exhibiting expanded noun phrases, prepositional phrases, indirect objects, and some coordinated sentences linked with *and* as well as some subordinate sentences. The child would be demonstrating evidence of copula, auxiliaries, pronouns, and the "ing," regular plural and regular past tense inflections. This is a general description for the oral language of a normal three-and-one-half-year-old child. A complete profile chart is available in Crystal, Fletcher, and Garman (1976, p. 106).

The child with language problems typical of their pattern one would present a profile like this at an older age. Crystal, Fletcher, and Garman suggest that enriched environment rather than language therapy seems to be indicated for these children. However, they do not indicate the extent of the age differential. We have seen children demonstrate a normal language pattern with a delay of one to three years. We maintain that the further in age the child is from the normal profile, the greater language problem this would present.

Patterns two to six were represented by the delayed language profiles and comprised the largest number of their cases. All of these patterns were represented by delays in syntactic development that were complicated by missing structures. The patterns are divided into separate specific problems at sentence/clause level and phrase level. As one might suppose, the patterns from two to six presented problems at increasing levels of sentence complexity. For example, cases with pattern two problems used oral language that consisted mainly of isolated words and a few phrases with an absence of sentences of any level. Crystal, Fletcher, and Garman said these were the most common cases.

Pattern three was apparent in problems with weak phrase structure. Sentences were simple. Pronouns were most often the subject and efforts to increase the use of definite and expanded noun phrases, subjects, or objects often result in breakdown of sentence structure.

Pattern four was represented by cases with reduced number of inflections (i.e. plural, past, comparative, possession) and a lack of compound words. These cases had satisfactory phrase and clause structure. Pattern five was the reverse of pattern four. These cases had strong word and inflectional patterns but weak phrase structure. In pattern six, complex sentence patterns or sentence connectivity were missing. The word level problems included problems of inflectional endings marking tense, number, comparatives, etc.

Pattern seven was typified by a profile with very limited utterances. While this sample seemed normal, no judgment could be made without further samples. However, nonverbal children were also included in this group.

Pattern eight was characterized by a profile that contained mostly deviant sentence types (i.e. "he want drink to") and some of the delayed types of patterns two to six.

Patterns nine to eleven were adult patterns. Patterns nine and ten were typically adult aphasic patterns and pattern eleven was represented by incomplete sentences.

While syntactic problems may vary, in general, a problem of syntax will be represented by ordering of the elements of a phrase, sentence, or discourse as well as the syntactic markers for number (singular versus plural), tense (regular and irregular past tense verbs), and comparative (adjectives—good/better/best).

The reader should be cautioned against developing presuppositions about any specific child's syntax before a careful individual analysis is made. Since the normal child's language may be individualistic, it stands to reason that the disordered child's language may be also quite individualistic.

Phonological Problems

The child with a disorder of phonology has a problem with the sounds and sound sequences of a language. The child has a different sound system. For some time, speech clinicians have lumped all of these problems under articulatory problems.

The distinction between an articulatory problem and a phonological problem may not always be clear. An articulatory problem should include an inability to produce a sound. The phonological problem should be represented by a different rule system for sounds and sound sequences. The confusion comes when a child does not produce a certain sound in his language—for instance an /s/. Does he never use the sound because he has never learned to produce such a sound or because he is unable to produce the sound, or does he not use the sound because this sound is not part of his phonological system or rules? This type of problem is open to both kinds of analysis and may in fact be a combination of problems. Perhaps at one time he was unable to produce an /s/ sound and thus he eliminated it from his language. It is easier to make a distinction in the case of a child with an inconsistent articulation error. Obviously this child can produce the sound; thus his problem becomes one of a different phonological sound system.

Compton (1975) expressed the view that the child with a phonological problem was not different from normal development but was presenting a "rigidity" system whereby the child retains earlier developmental patterns. Instead of dropping or replacing developmental sound substitutions or omissions, the child clings to them and makes them part of his linguistic system. Compton also noted the use of idiosyncratic sound patterns and thought that they may be caused by an attempt by the child to meet communicative needs.

The view that children with phonological disorders have sound patterns that are different from the norm but are consistent and analyzable in their own right, even if they are innovative, has begun appearing (Crocker, 1969; Compton, 1970, 1975; McReynolds and Huston, 1971; and Lorentz, 1976).

Lorentz (1976) expressed the position that most methods have analyzed individual needs and ignored the linguistic environment of the sounds. Lorentz postulates sets of phonological rules considering different contexts. His descriptions of underlying phonemic rules as well as surface phonetic constraints derived from transformations are a new addition to a description of phonological problems.

Compton (1976) has presented a phonological rule analysis method that seems easily useful in a clinical setting. He presented a detailed analysis of the phonological problems of a child called Grace (pp. 68-74). In order to demonstrate a phonological rule analysis, we have selected a few of these errors with the corresponding rule.

INITIAL DESCRIPTION

Underlying Sound	Child's Production	
	Initial position	*Final position*
/p/	[p] 2, [p =] 5	[p] 6
/t/	[t] 6, [t =] 9	[t] 8
/k/	[k] 4, [k =] 6	[k] 6

RULE

$$\begin{bmatrix} p \\ t \\ k \end{bmatrix} \rightarrow \begin{bmatrix} p = \\ t = \\ k = \end{bmatrix} \qquad /\#\underline{\quad\quad} \text{opt. } 60\%$$

This rule says that /p, t, k/ are produced nonaspirated at the beginning of a word (= denotes the sounds are unaspirated, # is linguistic boundary mark showing word beginning) optionally 60 percent of the time. The optional rule indicates that he produces these sounds some other way at other times. In this case, these sounds were appropriate in the remaining uses. The 60 percent is based on the proportionate frequency of occurrence in the sample.

Another phonological difference in Grace's sample is an error familiar to most speech clinicians.

INITIAL DESCRIPTION

Underlying Sound	Child's Production	
	Initial position	*Final position*
/θ/	[f] 4	[f] 8
/ð/	[d] 5	[v] 4

RULES

$$[\theta] \rightarrow [f] \qquad \begin{array}{l} /\#\text{——} \quad \text{oblig.} \\ /\text{——}r \quad \text{oblig.} \end{array}$$

$$[\eth] \rightarrow [d] \qquad /\#\text{——} \quad \text{oblig.}$$

$$\begin{bmatrix} \theta \\ \eth \end{bmatrix} \rightarrow \begin{bmatrix} f \\ v \end{bmatrix} \qquad /\text{——}\,\#\ \text{oblig.}$$

These rules specify that /f/ is substituted for /θ/ all the time (obligatory) in the initial position of a word both before a vowel and before the consonant /r/ in blends. Another substitution of /d/ for /ð/ is also used all the time (obligatory) in the initial position. The last rule specifies that /f/ is substituted for /θ/ and that /v/ is substituted for /ð/ obligatory in the final position of words.

These rules are not all-inclusive of Compton's phonological description of Grace's language but are presented as representative of the method of analysis by a rule system.

The descriptions of phonological problems are just appearing. Such late development is amazing considering the wealth of knowledge that has been available for some time about norms for articulatory development, and phonetic analysis of sounds as well as physiological and acoustic characteristics of speech. Ferguson and Garnica (1975) said, "It is possible to specify the child's phonological behavior with great precision. . . . This level of precision and theoretical insight is hard to match in other areas of child development. Moreover, the analysis of physiological development, more than other aspects of psycholinguistic research, seems to offer immediate promise for speech therapists and students of Speech Pathology, since in phonology the abnormalities can often be specified most unequivocally and therapeutic techniques tested most directly" (p. 154).

Pragmatic Problems

Pragmatics refers to the use of language in the social context. Pragmatics is an analysis of language that is independent of the grammar. Herriot (1970) suggested that we may find that pragmatic expectations may apply more to how one interprets a sentence than semantic rules.

Pragmatic rules then will of course refer to social conversational postulates and the intent to communicate in real life situations. The pragmatic rules include performatives, propositions, and presuppositions. The performatives are rules pertaining to the intent to communicate and include the speaker's goal in talking as well as the planned or unplanned result of the conversation. New words to describe the speech act performatives are locutionary acts (the actual sounds), illocutionary acts (the social act recognized by speaker and hearer) and perlocutionary acts (planned or unplanned effect created by the speaker). Proposition rules concern the common content of a sentence, and presupposition rules describe information that is not explicit in the utterance per se, but which must be understood by speaker and listener if the message is to be communicated.

Because pragmatic rules extend beyond the grammar they are often difficult to perceive. An example may help. Suppose you pass a person on the street and he says, "How are you?" Both speaker and hearer usually understand that as a greeting and not as an information seeking question. A caller on the phone who says, "Is Sue there?" means "May I speak to Sue?" Pragmatics then moves away from the literal interpretations of a sentence or sentences.

In the area of children's language this is the newest frontier. The work on normal development of Bates and her fellow researchers (Bates, Camaioni, and Volterra, 1975; Bates, 1976a, 1976b) stands nearly alone. The study of pragmatic disorders (Snyder, 1975; Rees, 1978) has been exploratory but has concluded with a hypothesis that children have trouble with pragmatic rules in early communication as well as with content later.

In the initial stages of considering pragmatic analysis of the oral language of a language impaired child at eight-and-one-half years, Bates and Johnston (1977) reported some examples. Among the conversational postulates, they noted that the child changed the topic frequently and did not follow topic ideas, that he was an unreliable informant, and that the amount of information he gave was poor. They also considered grammatical forms with pragmatic relevance, and observed simple use of articles and that the majority of nouns were unmarked for definiteness or were marked solely by possessives. More than half of his adjectives were possessives. Among the speech acts in major function of his discourse were questions or declaratives but imperatives, questions, and declaratives are usually present in equal proportions. He also left *yes/no* and *wh* questions unacknowledged. This is not an inclusive report of the Bates and Johnston analysis but is representative of the types of pragmatic language analysis explorations now being undertaken with children with language problems.

The types of problems that children may demonstrate are cognitive, semantic, syntactic, phonologic, and pragmatic. To have presented these separately and dichotomized has seemed necessary for purposes of clarity. Although these types of problems may exist in combination as well as separately, the more severe the language problem, the more likely the description of that problem will include problems from many areas.

CHILD GROUPINGS

Another facet that the speech clinician must be concerned with is the type of child who has the problem. Many of the children with language problems demonstrate neurological, physiological, mental, or emotional symptoms that fit a particular syndrome or type of child. In the past, these groups have been used as a label for the language problem. These children may have any or all of the before mentioned problems but as a group they are not a name of a problem. These groups are often called an etiological *label* of the problem. To state a causal factor of a language problem is usually presumptive and often unproveable; however, certain processing problems that frequently accompany etiologies may have an indirect, or perhaps even a direct, influence on language (for example, cognitive deficits are always accompanied by some kinds of language deficits). Regardless of this, to label the type of syndrome the child fits within does nothing to describe the language problem. We encourage a description of the problem and a description of other behaviors or history that describe the child and contribute to treatment. The following groups are presented in order to provide a description of children who may have a language problem. Any discussion of language problems within a particular group of children is presented in a very general manner. Because these children are individuals they may have any language problem and to presume specific problems particular to a type of child would do any child or diagnostic system a disservice.

Basically Normal

There is such an entity as a group of children who seem normal except for an existing language problem. These children have at least average intelligence. Physical and neurological evaluations indicate no problems. Hearing thresholds are within normal limits. Psychological tests or observations reveal no problems. The developmental history of these children indicates normal development and the home environment seems to present no problem. These children have an unremarkable history except that they do have a language problem. The language problem is usually one of oral performance and most of them comprehend well. In addition, they may show frustration when they want to communicate. These children seem normal except for a language problem. It seems fruitless to discuss the possibility that some undetermined problem is present. Of course, that possibility exists, but to date evidence has not been discovered supporting that view.

Very little has appeared in print concerning the basically normal child with a language problem. Only in recent years have authors begun to note that such a child exists. Yet, T. T. S. Ingram (1975) said that 30 to 40 percent of children seen in hospital speech clinics are basically normal children except that they have problems with spoken language. If the group is this large, it is amazing so little has appeared in writing about them.

The oral language of these children is usually described as following the developmental sequence but like that of a younger normal language child. T. T. S. Ingram (1975), B. Brown (1976), and Willbrand (1977b) reported delayed onset of speech; Ingram said that many of the children came from families with a history of delayed onset of oral language. Specific language problems of this group of children have been noted. Ingram said most of the children had phonological problems.

Willbrand reported problems in combining words at the two-word utterance level. Menyuk and Looney (1972) noted syntactic problems at the early sentence level. They demonstrated that on a repetition-of-sentence test the children with language problems (mean chronological age 6.2) had greater difficulty with all sentence types than children with normal language development (mean chronological age 4.6).

Further analysis of the oral language problems remains to be made. Obviously missing is any information about what happens to these children as they get older—do they eventually catch up, do they remain slightly delayed, or do they get further and further behind?

B. Brown (1976) observed that, in common with children with normal language, apparently normal children with language problems have individual language strategies. That means that the individual strategies for language acquisition or use will need to be discovered in order to provide adequate treatment.

Environmentally Different

By the middle 1960s the view that children who had been considered disadvantaged, deficient, or substandard in their use of language should be regarded as different language users emerged. This movement was primarily headed by sociolinguists who took the position that while the language the children used might indeed be different from the white, middle-class language of the American school system, their language was equally rich, structured, and acceptable within their own language community. Detailed discussions of this changing perspective are available in Williams (1970).

This movement was furthered by research in black English. Grammar rules of black English (not necessarily indicating that if one's skin color is black one must use black English) appeared as well as studies of the language differences of black children. The black English research (Stoller, 1975; Bentley and Crawford, 1973) doubtlessly contributed the driving force relative to the changing theoretical positions that different is not deficient. While other language differences such as those demonstrated by Mexican Americans, native Americans, and various Oriental groups have not been equally researched, some literature is beginning to emerge.

In order to understand what we mean by a different language, consider some of the rules of black English that are different from standard English. In phonology, for example, the voiced /ð/ in standard English changes in black English. In the initial position it becomes /d/ so that *this, that, these,* and *they* are expressed as *dis, dat, dese,* and *dey*. In the medial and final position, it usually is a /v/ sound so that *brother* is *brover* and *bathe* is *bave*. The voiceless *th* of standard English is different in black English also. In the initial position, the /t/ sound is usually used so that *thought* is *tought*. Since /d/ is substituted for /ð/, we would expect /t/ to be used in place of /θ/; however, if /θ/ is followed by an /r/, we might expect an /f/ sound so that *through* becomes *frough*. In the medial position, /f/ is the most frequently used sound so that *birthday* is *birfday, nothing* is *nofing,* and /f/ is usually the choice instead of the final voiceless *th* as in *toof* instead of *tooth*.

In syntax many of the differences center around the verbs. For instance, the statement "he is here all the time" to express continuing action in black English is expressed by use of *be* as in "he be here," and the negation of black English, "I don't got none" is different from "I don't have any." If we consider the sentence "John he over to his friend house," we could observe the difference in subject expression, in preposition, and in the possessive marker. These few examples are presented in order to give the reader an idea of the differences we are discussing, not to present the entire spectrum of differences. More complete discussions of the rule differences are available elsewhere (see for instance Fasold and Wolfram, 1975; Baratz, 1970; and Chapter 1 of this book).

The question for the speech clinician is usually whether a child's language use is reflective of a difference or of a disorder. Yoder (1970) suggested that the guideline to use was whether or not the child was using language appropriate in his given speech community. If the child's language was acceptable in his own language community then he is displaying a language difference. If the child does not function within the norms of any language community then he has a language disorder. For distinguishing characteristics of difference versus disorder see Williams and Wolfram (1977). Further discussion on how one may attempt to differentiate this will be found in Chapter 3.

A view such as this implies several things. First, any clinician working in an area where children demonstrate language difference, whether they are Appalachian, Chicano, or inner-city white, will have to know the language system of that community. Secondly, although a child has a language difference, he may also have a language disorder. Language disorders among the language different population may be in about the same proportion as among the normal population, but we have no research evidence to demonstrate that.

Certainly the speech clinician must be able to treat the disorders of language among any group, but a debatable issue is whether the clinician should treat a language difference. If we assume the position that regardless of the quality of the difference, the people who want to change their status, pursue higher education, or assume better employment will have to also learn the language of the mass—standard English—(for a review of this position see Stoller, 1975 and Fishman, 1973), then we must grapple with the problem of who should teach standard English. It seems logical to assume that a speech clinician would assume part of that responsibility. If we are teaching standard English, we are not correcting a disorder and the approach must be different. Another aspect of the problem of the environmentally different child might be poverty.

Environmentally Disadvantaged

The term disadvantaged has recently seemed to have negative connotations. This may have stemmed in part from the descriptions of disadvantaged children offered by authors such as Bereiter and Englemann (1966) who purported that retardation was the intellectual status of these children and that lack of verbal learning was an outstanding characteristic. Since sociolinguistics presented the concept of different, the term disadvantaged has seemed distasteful.

On the other hand, some researchers would agree that the problems of low socioeconomic families have presented some special concomitants to language problems. The currently popular term seems to be poverty children. We have separated the discussion of poverty children from the environmentally different to indicate that the possible effects of poverty on language may involve children speaking standard English as well as different language patterns.

In most discussions poverty children are determined by some level of low family income. While this arbitrary level may be a general guideline, it may also be misleading. We have seen children from farm families in the midwest who were classified as disadvantaged children on the basis of family income and yet the children were not educationally, linguistically, or socially disadvantaged. As long as we recognize the fallacy of the arbitrary family income level specifying a poverty child, we can proceed to present some of the general problems omitting the discussion of language differences.

Anastasiow and Hanes (1976), presenting a behavioristic view, stressed that parents of a poverty child do not emphasize aspects of communication such as reasoning, achievement standards, and reward systems that are necessary for success in school. They also believe that the poverty child has not had "experience" with language; that is, the lower class parents have not expanded the children's utterances in early language years or have not encouraged the child to be novel and play with language. For instance, "Silly, nilly, Willy, Billy, hilly," etc. (p. 55) were suggested as types of playing with language. They also stressed that poverty children have not been taught the importance of success in school nor the eagerness in quest of knowledge nor the need to cooperate with adult requests.

However, one of the problems with the compliance with requests may be the difference in the linguistic code. Bernstein (1970) talks of the difference in the communication code of poverty families. Unfortunately he used the label "restricted code" to apply to the code used by low-income families and "elaborated code" to label the code of middle-class families. He used the terms to point out cultural differences and not to specify poor versus good language. The restricted code of the lower class is much more rigid and demonstrates less variety in syntactic alternatives. Vocabulary selection is not a distinguishing factor.

Bernstein points out the different modes of social control. For instance, the restricted code tends to rely on imperative controls of behavior (i.e. "shut up," "get out") in which the child responds to external control and is not encouraged or offered explanations that allow him to internalize his own rules. He further elaborates this external control by talking about the positional appeal of the restricted code ("children kiss their grandpa," p. 43) versus the personal appeal of the elaborated code ("I know you don't like kissing grandpa, but he is unwell and he is very fond of you, and it makes him very happy." p. 45).

Bernstein elaborates his position further by considering how the lack of internalizing and personal problem solving places the child attending middle-class schools at a disadvantage. Another problem presented by Bernstein (1972) is that the development of personal values and setting of future rewards are not existent in lower socioeconomic groups but are necessary for success in school. The lower class child tends to respond descriptively and with little sense of any time but the present.

While some of the views expand the idea of the communication problems of poverty children, the environmental disadvantaged may be found in unexpected places. We are reminded of a four-year-old, nonverbal, cerebral palsied child. After some investigation, we discovered that this clean, neat child, seemingly well kept and loved, had spent nearly every waking hour tied to a chair in front of the television. In this manner the parents could be sure the child would be entertained but would not fall and hurt herself. She had never been allowed to crawl or walk with support and explore her home environment. She had never seen herself in a mirror or been allowed to eat with other people. She had never been outside to play in the grass, touch a flower, play with children, or go to town or to any store. The only time she got out of the house was to be carried to the car and then into the cerebral palsy center where she began her education at four years.

In our view this handicapped child from a middle-class home was environmentally disadvantaged. The clinician should not look for disadvantaged children only among poverty children.

From the above discussion, one would logically conclude that poverty, as such, has a direct and uncontaminated influence upon language development and academic achievement. A precaution needs to be included; it has been demonstrated that the incidence of nutritional and health problems is very high in poverty populations, including central nervous system impairment, hearing impairments, etc. (Tjossem, 1976). It therefore becomes somewhat presumptuous to assume other than a complex interaction of poverty and other related variables with disordered language.

Hearing Handicapped

Children with a hearing handicap have a hearing loss to such an extent that the loss interferes with educational and social interaction. The child is usually considered deaf when conversational speech is not understood. When the hearing loss is congenital or acquired in as early as the first three years of life, the result is a major handicap in communication. Oral language is the major area of handicap for the child. By the very nature of deafness, the child has little or no access to spoken language and consequently the entire process of normal language acquisition is impeded. This language problem underlies insufficiencies in other areas and is the most salient differentiating factor between a hearing child and a deaf child with the single handicap of hearing loss. It stands to reason that impeded reception of language will result in impeded acquisition of oral language use (Tracy, 1962; DiCarlo, 1964; Vernon, 1969; Moores, 1970; Brennan, 1975).

Given the current belief that normal children possess an innate capacity for language acquisition, it may be assumed that children without hearing still have this system innately specified, providing that the deafness is not the result of brain damage. It is not the case that they are incapable of processing the language data, the problem is one of receiving the primary data that is the language from their environment so they may establish their own repertoire of novel utterances based on a system of rules (Moores, 1970; Brennan, 1975).

While most of the studies in the language of hearing impaired children have concentrated on sign language, a few current studies are reporting information about the oral language of these children. While deaf children begin cooing and babbling at the same time normal children do, by about six months differences in the deaf child's repertoire of sounds become apparent (Miller, 1954; Lenneberg, 1967; Eisenson, 1972). This babbling stage continues in the deaf child through the early childhood years.

The deaf child seems to acquire a language code in the same order as hearing children, but at a much slower rate (Simmons-Martin, 1972). Some disagreement exists concerning how much slower the rate is. The disagreement may be due to the differing abilities of the children studied. DiCarlo (1964) said that a five-year-old deaf child would probably have a single-word vocabulary of less than 25 words. D. M. Dale (1974) said that by five years, 250 words would be excellent development and that most of those words would be used as single-word utterances. Griswold and Commings (1974) studied deaf children from one-and-a-half to three years of age and reported smaller vocabularies than normal children, but their subjects were talking in these years. They reported that the children were mainly using nouns, but they were also using modifiers, pronouns, verbs, and prepositions.

In a study of one child at four years of age (West and Weber, 1974), the child was using single words as well as two-word utterances—somewhat typical of stages described by pivot grammar or semantic analyses.

It seems the deaf child will begin onset of language from a year to four years behind the normal hearing child. While the subsequent stages seem to be about the same as for a normal child, hearing impaired children do not progress at the same rate of syntactic growth in comparison with chronological age increases as do normal children (Presnell, 1973).

As these children get older, their oral language begins to be different; whether this different language is the result of the hearing loss or the result of teaching might remain an unanswered question. By thirteen years of age, the hearing impaired adolescent is not using main verbs correctly (Presnell, 1973) and is substituting, adding, and omitting elements in the word order of sentences (Brannon and Murray, 1966). In general these teen-agers used simple active declarative sentences of the subject + verb + object type. They use few words to expand sentences other than *and* or *because* or occasionally *while* (Brannon and Murray, 1975; Goda, 1964).

The language problems of the hearing impaired child might also be complicated by the effects of an additional handicap.

Minimum Cerebral Dysfunction

Minimum cerebral dysfunction or minimal brain dysfunction is a medical label usually based on behavioral characteristics (Wender, 1971). No speech clinician should ever label a child as having a minimal cerebral dysfunction because such a label infers a medical diagnosis. However, it is well to be aware of the behavioral characteristics that contribute to such a diagnosis.

Kirk (1972) explained that in minimal cerebral dysfunction a neurologist does not usually find definite indications of damage but has to infer the damage from the behavioral signs. The soft neurological signs generally are described as including mild impairment of fine motor movement or coordination, problems in attention and activity, specific memory or perceptual deficits, and emotional lability. To this generally used description, Lerner (1976) adds delayed speech development as another soft sign.

If children exhibiting these characteristics are identified at an early age, minimal cerebral dysfunction is usually the medical term that is used. Freston (1972) says the term is used to indicate that central nervous system dysfunction is thought to cause learning disorders. Educators seem to think there is little educational benefit to infer cerebral dysfunction from behavior (Kirk, 1972).

Certainly the educational label for these children is "learning disability," but a child cannot be diagnosed as having a learning disability with certainty until he is about seven years of age. Public Law 93-380 specifies the connection between minimal cerebral dysfunction and learning disability and further defines the child in educational terms as follows: "Three characteristics common to all minimal cerebral dysfunctioning (learning disabled) children are average or above average intelligence, accurate sensory acuity, and achievement that is less than the composite of their intelligence, age, and educational opportunity would predict."

In addition to the notation of a specific learning disability in the presence of at least average intelligence and hearing and vision acuity, others would more specifically indicate that a learning disability is a language disability. This definite connection is stated in the Learning Disabilities Act of 1969 (cited in Kirk, 1972, pp. 43-44). "Children with special (specific) learning disabilities exhibit a disorder in one or more of the basic psychological processes involved in understanding or in using spoken or written language. These may be manifested in disorders of listening, thinking, talking, reading, writing, spelling or arithmetic."

The specific oral language problems have been included, problems in comprehension (Chalfant and Scheffelin, 1969; Lapointe, 1976) as well as word retrieval, syntax, and semantics (McLoughlin and Wallace, 1975). As the children become adolescents, the syntactic problems remain obvious (Lapointe, 1976; Wiig, 1976).

Central Nervous System (CNS) Impaired Children

Although the involvement of the central nervous system is only implied in children with minimal cerebral dysfunction and is based primarily upon "soft" or indirect signs, numerous children will be encountered by the speech pathologist who have known central nervous system impairment based upon "hard" or observable neurological signs. The likelihood that these children will become part of the caseload of the speech pathologist is substantially increasing as a consequence of the passage of the Education of All Handicapped Children Act of 1975.* The major hard signs of central nervous system impairment discussed in this section are mental retardation (moderate, severe, and profound), cerebral palsy, and congenital blindness-deafness (usually, but not always, the sign of central nervous system impairment). Grouping these children under the general class of CNS impair-

---

* This act mandates that educational programs shall be made available to *all* handicapped children between the ages of six and eighteen, and hopefully will be made available to all handicapped children ages three through five and nineteen through twenty-one.

ment for purposes of educational programming is facilitative since they share multiple problems that can be best handled by a team of specialists working in some coordinated fashion. For example, the physical therapist is primarily responsible for planning and implementing programs for development of neuro-motor posturing and ambulation; the occupational therapist is primarily responsible for planning and implementing programs for development of self-help skills, such as feeding, undressing and dressing, grooming, and simple housekeeping activities; the audiologist is primarily responsible for auditory evaluation and hearing training; and the speech pathologist is primarily responsible for planning and implementing programs for improving communicative skills, which include such things as language, voice, articulation and discrimination, etc. One cardinal rule, however, for dealing with severely handicapped children with CNS impairment is that the intervention program for these children cannot be fractionated, i.e. various specialized services cannot be planned and administered as separate and autonomous programs for a given child. All team members must be involved in the joint evaluation, planning, and implementation of all program objectives for a given child, and all must be aware of where the child is in a program, and what particular skills are being achieved over the total program spectrum at any given time. It therefore behooves the speech pathologist to not only be aware of problems that have traditionally been considered the province of other specialists, but to know something about the planning and implementation of the total program for the child. More will be said about this integrated team approach to planning and intervention in the chapter on remedial procedures.

"*Information processing models* have proven tremendously useful as a research tool in helping to understand many of the behavioral phenomenon that characterizes the areas of perception, learning, memory and language. In general, cognitive information-processing models include: (1) a stage of sensory information store, a high capacity storage system from which information rapidly decays but from which selected elements are recorded and transferred to the second stage, (2) short-term memory, or short-term store, a temporary holding area where information is maintained for immediate use or supported, for example, by rehearsal, and transferred for entry into, (3) long-term store, from which information is retrieved on subsequent occasions" (Ross and Leavitt, 1976, p. 112).

Since the brain is the primary organ for receiving, comprehending, formulating, and producing language, it follows that brain impairment is likely to have a direct effect upon these processing functions, although factors other than brain impairment may also have an interfering effect. The remaining part of this section will address itself to some general descriptions of language processing deficits of CNS impaired children and, in a general way, describe some of the language problems that may be encountered.

ATTENTIONAL DEFICITS. Many CNS impaired children do not seem to be able to attend to nearly as large a number of simultaneous stimuli as nonimpaired children (Wilhelm and Lovaas, 1976). This results in an overselectivity or narrowing of the number of features that can be processed simultaneously or in rapid sequence. In many severely mentally retarded children, orientation or attentional reactions are difficult to evoke, regardless of the strength of the stimulus material; with others orientation reaction (OR) is maximized upon the slightest stimulation and is difficult to suppress well enough for either paired-associate or serial learning to take place (Luria, 1963). The role played by the process called attention is at this date still rather opaque, especially as that role may relate to language problems. A number of studies, however, have shown that ability to optimize an attentional posture toward incoming stimuli plays a very important role in momentary sensory storage, discrimination, and recognition of both verbal stimuli (Loftus and Loftus, 1976; Krupski, 1977; Dorry, 1976) and nonverbal stimuli (Zeaman and House, 1963).

A recent series of studies (Tallal and Piercy, 1973a, 1973b, 1974, 1975; Tallal, Stark, and Curtiss, 1976; Tallal and Newcomb, 1978) have strongly suggested that a certain group of borderline CNS (often called dysphasic) children and aphasic adults have a similar difficulty in processing rapidly changing acoustic stimuli. If acoustic-stimulus changes require a formant transition period of 43 msec or less, dysphasic children have great difficulty learning to differentiate between them. If the same acoustic-stimulus changes require a formant transition no faster than 95 msec, the dysphasic children in the studies could differentiate as well as the normal control subjects. These findings tend to support the notion that dysphasic children are primarily impaired in auditory temporal processing and that this problem may have a debilitating effect upon their language comprehension. In one study, Tallal, Stark, and Curtiss (1976) had dysphasic children between the ages of seven and nine-and-one-half years imitate nonsense (V, CV, and CVC) syllables and name pictures spontaneously, and analyzed their syllabic production errors. Since the dysphasic children's perceptual errors had been found to be proportional to rapidity of change of critical formants, it was speculated that these children's production errors would be progressively greater with phonemes whose contexts created progressively shorter formant durations. Although the results were not clear cut, there was a tendency for production errors to be related to rapidity of change in formants of the produced phonemes. The Tallal et al. studies found the perceptual processing difficulties with rapidly changing acoustic stimuli to be one of the most salient perceptual problems of dysphasic children and adults, and virtually absent in normal children and adults.

Other studies have also supported the notion that dysphasic children have difficulty in processing for auditory recognition and discrimination of rapidly occurring acoustic verbal stimuli (Lowe and Campbell, 1965; Furth and Pufall, 1966; May, 1967; Stark, 1967; Rosenthal, 1970; Weiner, 1972; Eisenson, 1972). Although we do not know whether attentional disturbances are causal or only nosological in these auditory processing difficulties, we cannot help believing that ability to attend selectively may be a very important variable.

SHORT-TERM MEMORY DEFICITS. The length of time that information can be held in short-term memory (without recycling through the rehearsal process) has an upper limit of no more than fifteen seconds in normal adults (Loftus and Loftus, 1976). We also know that short-term memory is much shorter than this in very young children, gradually increasing with maturation.

We usually equate short-term memory with the ability to repeat strings of digits or words of varying lengths; this is the usual way of assessing short-term memory in children. However, in Chapter 1 we suggested that short-term memory could be broken into several component processes including short-term holding, imitation, organization (categorization, etc.), and rehearsal. If these particular processes are involved in handling verbal information—and introspection, logic, and a number of research studies (see Loftus and Loftus, 1976; Jenkins, 1973 for reviews) suggests that they are—we would expect that any involvement of these processes in the CNS impaired children would be detrimental to development of language facility. CNS impaired children do appear to be generally less capable of processing all components of short-term memory (Ellis, 1963, 1970; Kellas et al., 1973; Dugas, 1975; Luszcz and Bacharach, 1975; Ross and Leavitt, 1976). R. Brown (1973) has suggested that telegraphic speech was a reflection of various constraints in early language, one of which might be short memory span. There is also a growing belief that rehearsal strategies are an extremely important process in holding information for an indefinite time in short-term memory store and in transferring information into long-term store. CNS impaired children, as well as normal children with language delay, appear to be deficient in utilizing rehearsal strategies for language processing and retention (Allen, 1971; Kellas et al., 1973; Luszcz, 1975; Dugas, 1975). Much interest is being generated for future process oriented research in CNS impaired children.

LATERAL DOMINANCE FOR LANGUAGE FUNCTIONS. It is now rather common knowledge that the left hemisphere plays a more dominant role in handling the logical operations of language comprehension and production than the right one and that lateralization of left hemisphere dominance progresses gradually in the majority of children from equipotentiality in infancy to a high degree of left dominance by puberty (Zangwill, 1975; Lenneberg, 1975). It seems quite clear that there is an ontogenetic brain lateralization for linguistic (left) and nonlinguistic (right) dominance. The fact that lateralization of dominance is not as definite in many persons who have communicative disorders (Berry, 1969) creates an interest in the possible linkage of lateral dominance and reduced language ability. In spite of the fact that laterality and language relationships have been speculated about for decades, little, if any, research has been done with the CNS impaired population. If it were possible to show that children with reduced language ability also have reduced lateral dominance for language processing, the plausibility of functional interaction of these two variables might be strengthened. With the advent of techniques for assessing dominance in language processing through dichotic listing tests, it is now possible to analyze more precisely hemisphere dominance for language. A recent study of Down's syndrome children (Sommers and Starkey, 1977) suggests that severely language impaired children are less likely to show right ear advantages than are those with higher level language skills; this difference in ear advantage was not found to be related to mental age.

OTHER PROBLEMS IN LANGUAGE PROCESSING. Cromer (1974) found that mentally retarded children seem to differ somewhat from normal children in their strategies for learning certain rules that emerge at the upper bounds of the sensitivity or critical period for language learning; their strategies were centered around learning to use adjectives as cues for retrieving the deep meaning of a sentence pair such as "The duck is *easy* to bite." and "The duck is *willing* to bite." Normal children below the mental age of six years use a "primitive" interpretation, which usually depicts the object or unnamed noun as the recipient of the action. Not until age nine or ten are they able to understand the correct underlying meaning of these contrasting pairs. During the intermediate learning stage, the normals erroneously interpreted the adjectives as depicting the object nouns as recipients about 50 percent of the time and the subject noun as recipient about 50 percent of the time. However, the retarded subjects, chronological ages between fifteen to sixteen years, did not go through a stage of 50 percent strategy instability but rather used the primitive stage until they reached the stage of "correct" interpretation. Cromer suggests that this difference may be attributable to the relationship of the *sensitivity* period to the rule learning process, i.e. the retarded children may have passed beyond the period when they could make use of innate language-specific abilities in developing the adjective rules and thus must move directly from the primitive to the adult stage of competence.

Cromer suggests that the linguistic strategy of searching for the marked form of a linguistic structure is a critical period phenomenon and is lost to persons who pass the critical period without developing this strategy.

Guess and Baer (1973) were able to demonstrate that learning to encode and decode a linguistic form may be nosological rather than interdependent. When mentally retarded subjects were trained to understand or use a form, there was little generalization from use to comprehension or vice versa. This is an interesting finding that needs additional investigation.

Frith and Frith (1974) compared Down's syndrome children, autistic children, and normals on a simple tapping task and motoric tracking task. Only the Down's syndrome subjects did not improve with rest periods. A number of studies have indicated that the imitation ability of Down's children is superior to their spontaneous productions. This suggests that short-term memory for handling feedback is superior to long-term memory for motor planning.

Literature has frequently reported that some mentally retarded children manifest an astounding ability to memorize adult-like vernacular with a precocious vocabulary (often in the form of television commercials), but are unable to communicate their own independent ideas (Lillywhite and Bradley, 1969). Yet no specific data seem to be available to verify this concept. Hydrocephalic children are often described as superfluent (Cromer, 1974; Schwartz, 1974). Fleming (1969) collected speech samples from eleven hydrocephalic children; their CAs ranged from four to eight years and their IQs ranged from 73 to 101. He found that their verbal output was not significantly different from expectations at various mental ages, but that there was a greater number of inappropriate or irrelevant responses than one would encounter in normal children. The problem of creative use of novel sentences for communication versus use of memorized, stereotyped, and conditioned phrases by children with various types of cognitive impairment needs to be more fully researched.

Lenneberg (1962) wrote a case report on an eight-year-old boy who showed extensive comprehension of English but could not produce any speech due to a congenital inability to acquire motor speech skills (anarthria), suggesting that language can develop in the absence of expressive realization.

Birch and Lefford (1964) found cerebral palsied children less capable of integrating information coming in through two or more modalities than normal children.

Because these studies give us only bits and pieces of fragmentary information on various language processing problems in CNS impaired children, it is not possible to draw any systematic conclusions. It would probably be helpful to use some kind of processing model (perhaps like the one suggested in Chapter 1) as a basis of study, including evaluation and planning, relative to processing impairments and language in CNS impaired children.

LANGUAGE COMPREHENSION AND PRODUCTION. There have been a number of studies that depict mentally retarded children as being quantitatively delayed rather than qualitatively different from normal children in their language development. Karlin and Strazzulla (1952), Graham and Graham (1971), Byrne (1959), Morehead (1975), and Wheldall (1976) report that language development seems to have a higher dependence on mental age progression and cognitive development than any other variables and that language seems to follow normal patterns of development but at a slower rate.

PHONOLOGY. Information on phonological errors of mentally retarded children is relatively sketchy since it has become available mostly as a by-product of studies devoted primarily to analysis of articulation errors (Irwin, 1942, 1972; Bangs, 1942; Karlin and Strazulla, 1952; and Schlanger, 1953a, 1953b; etc.). Available information suggests that mentally retarded subjects acquire phonological skills in a normal but greatly delayed fashion; they also display an abnormal persistence in some of the common errors found in early speech patterns of normal children; mentally retarded children are much like other deviant children (D. Ingram, 1976) in that their normal acquisition stages are compounded by a perseveration of earlier stages, making their phonological picture seem very complex. Although these studies have shown articulation development to be comparable to expectations for various mental ages, there is no reliable data to show how phonological development relates to mental age; it seems logical, however, to assume there is a positive relationship.

Phonological errors of moderately retarded children tend to be similar in frequency and type to those found in younger children, with substitutions predominating. However, severely retarded tend to have a greater number of deletions and, in that sense, differ from the usual developmental pattern (Irwin, 1972).

Bodine (1974) studied the phonological development of two mongoloid children. His greatest obstacle with one of the children was that 67 percent of his utterances were unintelligible. The second child's speech was 75 percent intelligible and showed many of the phonological processes normal for younger children. Initial consonants were generally correct with a small number of substitutions. Voiced stops and fricatives were deleted—this appears to be an abnormal perseveration in view of the relative intactness of initial consonants and many consonant clusters. Both children showed abnormal persistence of certain phonological stages. Both children tended to use grunts, i.e. glottal stop plus an oral or nasal midfront or midcentral vowel, systematically as part of their communication; these were especially predominant (25 percent of utterances) in the severely delayed child.

Dodd (1975, 1976) compared the phonological rules of ten Down's syndrome children with those of ten normal children matched for mental age. She also compared non-Down's severely retarded with normal children matched for mental age. The Down's syndrome children phonological errors were more inconsistent than those of the normal children or non-Down's retarded children; some of their errors could not be accounted for by any phonological rules. The phonological errors of non-Down's syndrome retarded children corresponded more closely to those of the normal children than did those of the Down's syndrome children. Down's syndrome children were more prone to repeat syllables within a word, e.g. *meta-meta-mato* for *tomato* or *denten* for *dentist*. Some words were reduced to only vowel utterances, e.g. *e-e* for *elephant,* and in other words entire consonant clusters were omitted, e.g. *wi-ers* for *whiskers*. There were also many inconsistent phonological substitutions with up to as high as five phonemes being substituted at various times for one particular sound.

Dodd also found that repetition speech samples of the non-Down's retarded children and the normal children contained the same phonological errors as their spontaneous speech samples, but Down's syndrome children's repeated speech samples contained less phonological errors than their spontaneous speech samples. In a previous section on processes, it is speculated that the Down's syndrome children's short-term memory may be superior to their long-term memory for planning motor patterns; this could account for their superior phonological performance during repetition. The fact that they had mastered the same phonological rules as their normal and subnormal controls seems to rule out the possibility that the phonological differences are due to the inability of Down's syndrome children to acquire phonological rules (Cromer, 1974).

MORPHOLOGY. Lovell and Bradbury (1967) compared a large group of retarded children with the normative data of Berko (1958) on developmental morphology. They concluded that the retarded children could not generalize inflectional rules to new lexical items in obligatory contexts as well as normal children, even though the general mental-age level of the retarded group was higher than that of the normal children. It is possible that involvement of nonsense words could present a compounding problem for cognitively impaired children, especially if they have a tendency toward concrete orientation.

Newfield and Schlanger (1968), using the Berko test of morphological inflections, found that retarded children learn morphology in nearly identical order to normal children, although their rate of learning was slower. Both retarded and normal children learned regular and common allomorphs first. Both groups also did better in supplying morphological inflections to real words than to nonsense words. The retarded seemed less able to generalize from the familiar words to the nonsense words than the normal children. Dever and Gardner (1970) gave the same test to retarded children and found that they tended to give an incorrect response to nonsense words by repeating the word rather than generalizing the concept of adding the inflections.

Johnston and Schery (reported by Morehead, 1975) demonstrated that the phenomenon of ordinality of morpheme acquisition was not only similar for retarded and normal children, but also for other language deficient children.

Bradbury and Lunzer (1972) compared normal and subnormal children in their ability to learn universal versus dichotomous versus arbitrary rules for word inflection. In the universal rule, the same suffix (for example, *es*) was used with all ten nonsense words to designate a particular inflectional meaning (such as plural), while the dichotomous rule used two different suffixes (for example, *s* and *es*) each of which would designate the same inflectional meaning; in the arbitrary rule a different suffix was used with each of ten nonsense words but all ten suffixes designated the same inflectional meaning. The number of trials necessary for learning the universal rule was significantly less than the number necessary for learning the other two rules. The other two rules took about the same number of learning trials. The findings for both the normal and the subnormal children were identical. In another phase of their study, thirty new items were presented only once to assess transfer. The retarded subjects did more poorly than the normals in this phase of the study. It was not certain whether there was something about the single trial method with which the retarded have more trouble or whether the retarded were less willing to search through the use strategies available to them, e.g. rehearsal, when confronted with a single trial.

Dever (1972) has cautioned against placing too much confidence in generalizing formal test performance to the informal social context. His study showed that mentally retarded children's scores on the Berko test of morphology were not closely related to their use of English morphology in their natural environment.

SYNTAX. Lackner (1968) collected a language sample of 1,000

utterances from each of five retarded children ranging in mental ages from 2.3 to 8.8 years. The phrase structure grammar was written for each child and notation was made of transformations used. Comprehension and imitation of modified forms of the grammar of each child were assessed. Similar procedures were followed for five normal control children.

Lackner found that both normal and retarded children could understand and imitate any structure generated by rules at or below their level of grammatical development. Imitated sentences with a structure on a higher level than the grammatical levels of the children were modified by both normal and retarded subjects in such a way as to conform to rules on their level.*

Sentence lengths of the mentally retarded increased with mental age and were the same as for normal children at the same mental ages. Each phrase structure grammar at a particular mental age appeared to be a subset of the grammar at the next higher level.

Lackner found that sentence length of mentally retarded children with mental ages up to four-and-a-half were the same as for normal children at comparable chronological ages. However, sentence lengths of retarded children with mental ages beyond four-and-a-half were progressively less similar to those of normal children as ages increased. A very significant finding was the apparent invariance in the order of appearance of sentential types and phrase structure rules as mental age increases. Phrase structure grammar at each mental age level appeared to be a subset of the grammar at the next higher level. The number of transformations understood by the retarded children increased with increasing mental age.

Graham and Graham (1971) analyzed the syntax of nine non-mongoloid mentally retarded subjects in a state training school. The language samples were comprised of seventy-five sentences, and formulations of syntactic rules of each child were developed on the bases of the samples. All utterances could be rewritten in terms of a rather small number of phrase structure rules. A set

---

* For example, the sentence "Mary was hit by the ball" was repeated as "Mary ...hit...a...ball," "Mary...the...hit," and "Mary...ah...ball" respectively by three children who did not understand the sentence.

of transformational rules were then developed to allow recovery of the original surface structure. Two types of transformations were involved "(a) elementary transformations which resulted in changes in the underlying base strings through such operations as addition, deletion or substitution; (b) generalized transformations which acted on two (or more) underlying strings to produce a single derived structure through such operations as conjoining [e.g., 'Take the doll and put it on the table'] and embedding [e.g., 'He went to the store']" (Graham and Graham, 1971, p. 625).

There was a strong tendency for lower mental age subjects to utilize only base string rules with practically no transformations being applied. The tendency for higher mental age subjects tended to be just the opposite; the higher the mental age, the greater number of transformations were found per sentence. These tendencies were influenced by mental age but not chronological age. The conclusions reached by these investigators were similar to those reached by Lackner (1968); mental age appears to be an overriding factor and developmental rules used by retarded at given mental ages appear to be similar to those used by normal children at comparable chronological ages. No studies similar to these have been reported on Down's Syndrome children.

Bartel (1973) administered the Carrow Elicited Language Inventory to trainable children and compared their performance with normal children. When matched for mental age, the retarded children's use of lexical items did not differ from that of nonretarded children; however, use of grammatical categories by mentally retarded children was inferior to that of normal children of comparable mental age. Sentence comprehension by retarded children was found by Wheldall (1976) to be unaffected by social class while in a sample of normal children, social class had a very distinct effect. Wheldall speculated that retarded children did not benefit from the richer verbal environment of higher social classes due to inefficient incidental learning.

Some earlier studies on comprehension and imitation of sentences have suggested that severely retarded children have difficulty processing negation (Semmel and Greenough, 1971). Handling of the negative may be influenced by the possible ambiguity of the structures being negated. Lamberts and Weener (1976), for example, found that severely retarded children were able to correctly discriminate between two pictures—one in which a boy was flying a kite and another one in which a boy was sitting in a chair—when asked "Show me 'the boy is not flying a kite.' " but could not as readily discriminate between two pictures—one that showed a dog chasing a cat and another that showed a cat chasing a dog—when asked "Show me 'the dog is not chasing the cat.' " Lamberts and Weener concluded that reversibility of the sentence seems to affect the ease with which it could be comprehended, nonreversible ones being easier to comprehend than reversible ones.

Vocabulary. Mein and O'Connor (1960) analyzed 28,732 words of eighty retarded persons who were between ten and thirty years of age chronologically. Average size of expressive vocabularies of persons whose mental ages ranged from three to seven years was 106 to 677 words. This may be contrasted to an estimate of 34,000 words on the average for first-grade, middle-class normal children (Taylor and Swinney, 1972).

Beier et al. (1969) compared vocabulary usage of thirty mentally retarded subjects, ranging in IQ from 23 to 75 and in chronological age from eleven to twenty-four years, with that of normal children (12-16 years). All of the retarded subjects were male residents at the Utah State Training School who were known to be able to communicate intelligibly. No subjects suspected of being psychiatrically ill were included. A minimum of 2,700 words were elicited from each subject by an interviewer who asked open questions or suggested conversation topics. The responses of the subjects were recorded on tape for later counting and analysis.

Analysis of vocabulary usage was broken into the following types of counts: (1) average words per minute (WPM); (2) number of positive words, e.g. *yes, okay;* (3) number of negative words, e.g. *no, none;* (4) number of single self-reference words, e.g. *I, me, mine;* (5) number of plural self-reference words, e.g. *us, we;* and (6) number of question words. The mentally retarded subjects spoke significantly more slowly than normal subjects (60 WPM versus 172 WPM). The retarded subjects also used significantly more positive words than did normal controls. The mentally retarded group made less frequent reference to others and more frequent reference to themselves; the ten most frequently used words comprised a higher percentage of the total output than for normals. Type-token ratios (TTRs)* were also compared; the TTR of the retarded subjects differed significantly from that of normals, the TTR of normals being greater (suggesting a richer, more elaborate use of vocabulary). It was surprising to find that the TTR of the retarded with low IQs was greater than the TTR of those with higher IQs. Closer examination showed that the lower IQ subjects tended to use simpler sentence structure and devoted much of their time to enumerating many simple, grammatically unconnected words rather than to speaking in sentences, thus reducing the number of high frequency function words. This negative relationship between IQ and TTR in the retarded suggests that the lower IQ subjects are not as lacking in vocabulary as they are in conceptualization and more abstract rule learning. The excessive reference to "self" rather than to "others" may be used roughly as a predictor of immaturity. The lists of most frequently used words by both the normal and the mentally retarded subjects were fairly similar except for the excessive use of *I* by the retarded.

Anastasiow (1973) compared the responses of EMR children and their normal peers of varying chronological ages by means of a variation of the Menyuk repeated sentence task. He found EMRs to be similar to their chronological age peers on concrete word errors and similar to peers of a younger age on function word errors.

Spreen (1965) reported that Down's children use nouns significantly more often than other mentally subnormals. Normal children use more adjectives than nouns in picture descriptions, whereas for subnormals, nouns are used more frequently.

Emotionally Disturbed Children

The term *autism* is often used to describe an extreme form of emotional disturbance that is accompanied by language disorders.

---

* By definition, type-token ratio is the number of different words (types) used, divided by the total number of words (tokens) used.

In 1943 Leo Kanner published his first description of a syndrome that he called early infantile autism. Since then the term autism has become widely used, although sometimes differently used and frequently overused. Nevertheless, the syndrome is usually recognized as having the following clinical specificity: detachment from people, an obsessive desire for maintenance of sameness, a fascination with objects, and a failure to use language for communication. It is the language aspect of the problem that causes us to consider this specific syndrome. We do not encourage labeling all emotionally disturbed children as autistic.

Baltaxe and Simmon (1977) said that autistic children typically begin to develop verbally at a fairly normal rate during the first year-and-a-half, development decreases drastically from that point. Many authorities would use the label schizophrenia for children demonstrating this pattern and being diagnosed later. They did report that "language histories of autistic children show a considerable variability ranging from failure to develop communicative skills to delayed development or arrest after early normal development" (p. 376).

One of the major characteristics differentiating autistic children from other children is their increased quantity and different quality of use of imitation (echolalia). Baltaxe and Simmons (1975) reported that autistic children tend to imitate more frequently than normal children, and their imitations tend to be more exact replications of the adult model than those of normal children. A later report by them (Baltaxe and Simmons, 1977) cautions that one of the problems that renders this notion questionable is the apparent poor observer agreement as to what constitutes imitated rather than propositional speech.

It should be noted that about one third of these children remain mute, some autistic children speak once or twice in a lifetime, and some develop large vocabularies early. These large vocabularies consist mainly of naming things and/or delayed echolalia. They may be echoed immediately or stored and used later at inappropriate times. This vocabulary is seldom used to communicate. So in terms of real communication, the speaking child may be said to differ little from the mute child (Kanner, 1962).

In the children who do talk an unevenness of language maturity will be noted, but in general they can be compared to a child of a much younger age. For instance, the speech of an autistic child of seven might in some ways be compared with a normal child of two. The speech will be monotonous and characterized by very few questions, many repetitions of adults' phrases, incomplete sentences, and use of nouns for naming (Cunningham and Dixon, 1961).

Many other unusual things make the speech patterns more obvious. For instance, *yes* is a concept that takes an autistic child years to understand. Affirmation is characteristically indicated by the repetition of questions. For example, if he is asked, "Do you want an ice cream cone?" his affirmative indication that he does would be a response such as, "Do you want an ice cream cone?" (Kanner, 1944).

Speech is often characterized by literalness, such as the boy who was upset because his father talked of a picture *on* the wall rather than *near* the wall. There may be part-whole confusion, such as the boy who asked for dinner by saying, "Do you want some catsup, honey?" His favorite food was meat with catsup on it (Rimland, 1969, p. 15).

Since the autistic child has little or no desire to communicate, his language need not be the same as those in his environment. He may often coin words or expressions that have meaning only for him (neologisms) or he may have a language of his own (idioglossia) (Shirley, 1963).

Those who remain mute may in emergencies use good sentences with very clear meaning and then resume muteness, such as the mute five-year-old who had a prune skin stick to his palate. He became panicky and yelled, "Take it out of there!" and then resumed muteness (Kanner, 1949).

The ability of autistic children to label things seems to be much greater than their ability to recognize or use semantic-syntactic-relational constructions. A lack of use of past tense and pronouns (especially *I*) represent problems that seem to be more pronounced in autistic children than in normal children having approximately the same language age (Baltaxe and Simmons, 1975).

In their extended study of an eight-year-old autistic girl, using Weir's (1962) procedure for sampling the language of a normal two-and-a-half year old, Baltaxe and Simmons (1977) found that, like the normal child during early stages of verbal develop- ment, she seemed to take pleasure in sounds of language and in the playful manipulation of linguistic units. Unlike the normal child, however, she did not engage in dialogue with an imaginary interlocutor; this finding was congruous with earlier literature that has suggested that the autistic child seems unable to establish interpersonal relationships. Recurrences of a major theme were observed in the autistic child; these seemed to be similar to those described by Weir in normal subjects. She also tended to have a much greater number of ungrammatical utterances than would be expected of her general language level. Although she used the processes of expansion, substitution, and deletion in her construc- tions and put nouns, verbs, and modifiers in the correct slots, use of these transformational processes appeared to be different than one would expect from observing the normal child. They were stereotyped and often turned out to be ungrammatical when con- sideration was made of *contextual-sensitive* cues. Baltaxe and Simmons (1977) suggested that this is what one would expect to happen if language acquisition took place as a gradual breaking down of rote-learned echolalic patterns into individual chunks of varying sizes rather than as a gradually expanding system of linguistic categories and rules.

Although the study of language in autism is still in its infancy, as with other etiological groups, it appears to be another poten- tially rewarding area for future study.

SUMMARY

The present chapter has presented a summary of various lan- guage problems including cognitive, semantic, syntactic, phono- logic, and pragmatic disorders. It also describes various child- groupings that are currently receiving attention in the field of speech pathology and audiology—including basically normal, en- vironmentally different, emotionally disadvantaged, hearing handicapped, minimal cerebral dysfunctioning, central nervous system impaired, and emotionally disturbed children. The following chapters suggest various methods and techniques for measuring and evaluating language problems in these children.

References

Allen, J.: The effects of covert and overt rehearsal on children's imitation of meaningful and nonmeaningful speech. Unpublished master's thesis, University of Utah, Salt Lake City, 1971.

Anastasiow, N. J.: Miscue language patterns of mildly retarded and non-retarded students. *A J Ment Defic, 77:*431-434, 1973.

Anastasiow, N. J. and Hanes, M. L.: *Language patterns of poverty children.* Springfield: Thomas, 1976.

Baltaxe, C. and Simmons, J. Q.: Language in childhood psychosis. *J Speech Hear Disord, 40:*439-458, 1975.

Baltaxe, C. A. M. and Simmons, J. Q.: Bedtime soliloquies and linguistic competence in autism. *J Speech Hear Disord, 43:*373-393, 1977.

Bangs, J.: A clinical analysis of the articulatory defects of the feebleminded. *J Speech Hear Disord, 7:*343-356, 1942.

Baratz, J. C.: Teaching reading in an urban negro school system. In Williams, F. (Ed.): *Language and poverty.* Chicago: Markham, 1970.

Bartel, N.: Language comprehension in the moderately retarded child. *Exceptional Child, 30:*375-384, 1973.

Bates, E.: *Language and context: The acquisition of pragmatics.* New York: Acad Pr, 1976a.

Bates, E.: Pragmatics and sociolinguistics in child language. In Morehead, D. M. and Morehead, A. E. (Eds.): *Normal and deficient child language.* Baltimore, Maryland: Univ Park, 1976b.

Bates, E., Camaioni, L., and Volterra, V.: The acquisition of performatives prior to speech. *Merrill-Palmer Quarterly, 21:*205-226, 1975.

Bates, E. and Johnston, J. R.: Pragmatics in normal and deficient child language. Short course presented at the American Speech and Hearing Association convention, Chicago, November 1977.

Beier, E. G., Starkweather, J. A., and Lambert, M. J.: Vocabulary usage of mentally retarded children. *Am J Ment Defic, 73:*927-934, 1969.

Bentley, R. H. and Crawford, S. D.: *Black language reader.* Glenview, Illinois: Scott F, 1973.

Bereiter, C. and Engelmann, S.: *Teaching disadvantaged children in the preschool.* Englewood Cliffs, New Jersey: P-H, 1966.

Berko, J.: The child's learning of English morphology. *Word, 14:*150-177, 1958.

Bernstein, B.: A sociolinguistic approach to socialization: With some reference to educability. In Williams, F. (Ed.): *Language and poverty.* Chicago: Markham, 1970.

Bernstein, B.: Some sociological determinants of perception: An inquiry into sub-cultural differences. In Fishman, J. A. (Ed.): *Readings in the sociology of language*. Paris: Mouton, 1972.

Birch, M. F. and Lefford, A.: Two strategies for studying perception in brain-damaged children. In Birch, H. G. (Ed.): *Brain damage in children*. Baltimore, Maryland. Williams & Wilkins, 1964.

Bloom, L.: *Language development: Form and function in emerging grammars*. Cambridge, Massachusetts: MIT Pr, 1970.

Bodine, A.: A phonological analysis of the speech of two mongoloid (Down's syndrome) boys. *Anthropol Linguistics, 16*:1-24, 1974.

Bowerman, M.: Semantic factors in the acquisition of rules for word use and sentence construction. In Morehead, D. M. and Morehead, A. E. (Eds.): *Normal and deficient child language*. Baltimore, Maryland: Univ Park, 1976.

Bradbury, B. and Lunzer, E. A.: The learning of grammatical inflexions in normal and subnormal children. *J Child Psychol Psychiatry, 13*:239-248, 1972.

Brannon, J. B. and Murray, J.: The spoken syntax of normal, hard of hearing, and deaf children. *J Speech Hear Res, 9*:604-610, 1966.

Brennan, M.: Can deaf children acquire language? *Am Ann Deaf, 120*:463-479, 1975.

Brown, B. B.: Language vulnerability, speech delay and therapeutic intervention. *Br J Disord Commun, 11*:43-56, 1976.

Brown, R.: *A first language*. Cambridge, Massachusetts: Harvard U Pr, 1973.

Byrne, M. C.: Speech and language development of athetoid and spastic children. *J Speech Hear Disord, 24*:231-240, 1959.

Chalfant, J. C. and Scheffelin, M. A.: *Central processing dysfunctions in children*. Bethesda, Maryland: HEW, 1969.

Chappell, G. E.: Learning disabilities and the language clinicians. *J Learning Disabilities, 5*:610-619, 1972.

Chomsky, N.: *Syntactic structures*. Hague: Mouton, 1957.

Chomsky, N.: *Aspects of the theory of syntax*. Cambridge, Massachusetts: MIT Pr, 1965.

Compton, A. J.: Generative studies of children's phonological disorders. *J Speech Hear Disor, 35*:315-339, 1970.

Compton, J.: Generative studies of children's phonological disorders: A strategy of therapy. In Singh, S. (Ed.): *Measurement procedures in speech, hearing and language*. Baltimore, Maryland: Univ Park, 1975.

Compton, J.: Generative studies of children's phonological disorders: Clinical ramifications. In Morehead, D. M. and Morehead, A. E. (Eds.): *Normal and deficient child language*. Baltimore, Maryland: Univ Park, 1976.

Crocker, J. R.: A phonological model of children's articulation competence. *J Speech Hear Disord, 34*:203-213, 1969.

Cromer, R. F.: Receptive language in the mentally retarded: Processes and diagnostic distinctions. In Schiefelbusch, R. L. and Lloyd, L. L. (Eds.):

Language perspectives: Acquisition, retardation, and intervention. Baltimore, Maryland: Univ Park, 1974.

Cromer, R. F.: The cognitive hypothesis of language acquisition and its implications for child language deficiency. In Morehead, D. M. and Morehead, A. E. (Eds.): *Normal and deficient child language.* Baltimore, Maryland: Univ Park, 1976.

Crystal, D., Fletcher, P., and Garman, M.: *The grammatical analysis of language disability.* London: Edward Arnold, 1976.

Cunningham, M. and Dixon, C.: A study of the language of an autistic child. *J Child Psychol Psychiatry, 2:*193-202, 1961.

Dale, D.: *Language development in deaf and partially hearing children.* Springfield: Thomas, 1974.

Dale, P. S.: *Lanugage development: Structure and function* (2nd ed.). New York: HR & W, 1976.

Dever, R. B.: A comparison of the results of a revised version of Berko's test of morphology with free speech of mentally retarded children. *J Speech Hear Res, 15:*169-178, 1972.

Dever, R. B. and Gardner, W. I. Performance of normal and retarded boys on Berko's test of morphology. *Language and Speech, 13:*162-181, 1970.

DiCarlo, L. M.: *The deaf.* Englewood Cliffs, New Jersey: P-H, 1964.

Dodd, B.: Recognition and reproduction of words by Down's syndrome and non-Down's syndrome retarded children. *Am J Ment Defic, 80:*306-311, 1975.

Dodd, B.: A comparison of the phonological systems of mental-age matched, normal, severely subnormal and Down's syndrome children. *Br J Disord Commun, 11:*27-41, 1976.

Dorry, G. W.: Attentional model for the effectiveness of fading in training reading-vocabulary with retarded persons. *Am J Ment Defic, 81:*271-279, 1976.

Dugas, J.: Effects of stimulus familiarity on the rehearsal strategies transfer mechanism in retarded and non-retarded individuals. *Am J Ment Defic, 80:*349-356, 1975.

Eisenson, J.: *Aphasia in children.* New York: Har-Row, 1972.

Ellis, N. R.: The stimulus trace and behavioral inadequacy. In Ellis, N. R. (Ed.): *Handbook of mental deficiency.* New York: McGraw, 1963.

Ellis, N. R.: Memory processes in retardates and normals. In Ellis, N. R. (Ed.) *International review of research in mental retardation,* vol. 4. New York: Acad Pr, 1970.

Fasold, R. W. and Wolfram, W.: Some linguistic features of negro dialect. In Stoller, P. (Ed.): *Black American English.* New York: Dell, 1975.

Ferguson, C. A. and Garnica, O. K.: Theories of phonological development. In Lenneberg, E. H. and Lenneberg, E. (Eds.): *Foundation of language development,* vol. 1. New York: Acad Pr, 1975.

Fishman, J. A.: The sociology of language. In Miller, G. A. (Ed.): *Communication, language, and meaning.* New York: Basic, 1973.

Fleming, C. P.: The verbal behavior of hydrocephalic children. *Dev Med Child Neurol,* Supplement 15, pp. 74-82, 1969.

Freedman, P. P. and Carpenter, R. L.: Semantic relations used by normal and language impared children at stage I. *J Speech Hear Res, 19:*784-795, 1976.

Freston, C. W.: *Introduction to learning disabilities.* Unpublished manuscript. Available from Department of Special Education, University of Utah, Salt Lake City, 1972.

Frith, U. and Frith, C. D.: Specific motor disabilities in Down's syndrome. *J Child Psychol Psychiatry, 15:*293-301, 1974.

Furth, H. G. and Pufall, P. B.: Visual and auditory sequencing in hearing impaired children. *J Speech Hear Res, 9:*441-449, 1966.

Goda, S.: Spoken syntax of normal, deaf, and retarded adults. *J Verbal Learning and Verbal Behavior, 3:*401-405, 1964.

Graham, J. T. and Graham, L. W.: Language behavior of the mentally retarded: Syntactic characteristics. *Am J Ment Defic, 75:*623-629, 1971.

Griswold, E. and Commings, J.: The expressive vocabulary of pre-school deaf children. *Am Ann Deaf, 119:*16-28, 1974.

Guess, D. and Baer, D.: Some experimental analyses of linguistic development in institutionalized retarded children. In Lahey, B. (Ed.): *The modification of language behavior.* Springfield: Thomas, 1973.

Hannah, E. P.: *Applied linguistic analysis.* Northridge, California: Joyce, 1974.

Herriot, P.: *An introduction to the psychology of language.* London: Methuen, 1970.

Ingram, D.: *Phonological disability in children.* New York: Elsevier, 1976.

Ingram, T. T. S.: Speech disorders in childhood. In Lenneberg, E. H. and Lenneberg, E. (Eds.): *Foundations of language development,* vol. 2. New York: Acad Pr, 1975.

Irwin, O. C.: The developmental status of speech sounds of ten feeble-minded children. *Child Dev, 13:*29-39, 1942.

Irwin, O. C.: *Communication variables of cerebral palsied and mentally retarded children.* Springfield: Thomas, 1972.

Jenkins, J. J.: Language and memory. In Miller, G. A. (Ed.): *Communication, language and meaning.* New York: Basic, 1973.

Johnston, J. R. and Schery, T. K.: The use of grammatical morphemes by children with communication disorders. In Morehead, D. M. and Morehead, A. E. (Eds.): *Normal and deficient child language.* Baltimore, Maryland: Univ Park, 1976.

Kanner, L.: Autistic disturbances of affective contact. *Nervous Child, 2:*217-250, 1942-1943.

Kanner, L.: Early infantile autism. *J Pediatr, 25:*211-217, 1944.

Kanner, L.: Problems of nosology and psychodynamics of early infantile autisms. *Am J Orthopsychiatry, 19:*416-426, 1949.

Kanner, L.: *Child psychiatry,* 3rd ed. Springfield: Thomas, 1962.

Karlin, I. and Strazzulla, M.: Speech and language problems of mentally deficient children. *J Speech Hear Disord, 17:*286-294, 1952.

Kellas, G., Ashcraft, M. H., and Johnson, N. S.: Rehearsal processes in the short-term memory performance of mildly retarded adolescents. *A J Ment Defic, 77:*670-679, 1973.

Kirk, S. A.: *Educating exceptional children.* Boston: HM, 1972.

Krupski, A.: Role of attention in reaction-time performance of mentally retarded adolescents. *Am J Ment Defic, 82:*79-83, 1977.

Lackner, J.: A developmental study of language behavior in retarded children. *Neuropsychology, 6:*301-320, 1968.

Lamberts, F. and Weener, P. D.: TMR children's competence in processing negation. *A J Ment Defic, 81:*181-186, 1976.

Lapointe, C. M.: Token test performances by learning disabled and achieving adolescents. *Br J Disord Commun, 11:*121-133, 1976.

Lee, L.: Developmental sentence types: A method for comparing normal and deviant syntactic development. *J Speech Hear Disord, 31:*311-330, 1966.

Lenneberg, E. H.: Understanding language without ability to speak. *J Abnorm Social Psychol, 65:*419-425, 1962.

Lenneberg, E. H.: *Biological foundations of language.* New York: Wiley, 1967.

Lenneberg, E. H.: In search of a dynamic theory of aphasia. In Lenneberg, E. H. and Lenneberg, E. (Eds.): *Foundations of language development,* vol. 2. New York: Acad Pr, 1975.

Lenneberg, E. H., Nichols, I., and Rosenberger, E.: Primitive stages of language development in mongolism. *Disorders of Communication, 42:*119-137, 1964.

Lerner, J. W.: *Children with learning disabilities.* Boston: HM, 1976.

Lillywhite, H. S. and Bradley, D. P.: *Communication problems in mental retardation.* New York: Har-Row, 1969.

Loftus, G. R. and Loftus, E. F.: *Human memory: The processing of information.* New York: Wiley, 1976.

Lorentz, J. P.: An analysis of some deviant phonological rules of English. In Morehead, D. M. and Morehead, A. E. (Eds.): *Normal and deficient child language.* Baltimore, Maryland: Univ Park, 1976.

Lovell, K. and Bradbury, B.: The learning of English morphology in educationally subnormal special school children. *Am J Ment Defic, 71:*609-615, 1967.

Lowe, A. D. and Campbell, A. R.: Temporal discrimination in aphasoid and normal children. *J Speech Hear Res, 8:*313-314, 1965.

Luria, A. R.: *The mentally retarded child.* New York: Pergamon, 1963.

Luszcz, M. A. and Bacharach, V. R.: List organization and rehearsal instructions in recognition memory of retarded adults. *Am J Ment Defic, 80:*57-62, 1975.

MacDonald, J. D. and Blott, J. P.: Environmental language intervention: The rationale for a diagnostic and training strategy through rules, context, and generalization. *J Speech Hear Disord, 39:*244-256, 1974.

May, M. Z.: An experimental investigation of multimodal discrimination learning by aphasic children utilizing an automated apparatus. Unpublished doctoral dissertation, Stanford University, Stanford, California, 1967.

McLoughlin, J. A. and Wallace, G.: *Learning disabilities: Concepts and characteristics.* Columbus, Ohio: Merrill, 1975.

McReynolds, L. V. and Huston, K.: A distinctive feature analysis of children's misarticulations. *J Speech Hear Disord, 36:*155, 1971.

Mein, R. and O'Connor, N.: A study of the oral vocabularies of severely subnormal patients. *J Ment Defic Res, 4:*130-143, 1960.

Menyuk, P.: Comparison of grammar of children with functionally deviant and normal speech. *J Speech Hear Res, 7:*109-121, 1964.

Menyuk, P. and Looney, P. L.: A problem of language disorder: Length versus structure. *J Speech Hear Res, 15:*264-279, 1972.

Miller, G. A. and McNeill, D.: Psycholinguistics. In Lindzey, G. and Aronson, E. (Eds.): *The handbook of social psychology.* Reading, Massachusetts: A-W, 1969.

Miller, J.: Vocabulary needs of the preschool deaf child. *Volta Review, 56:*58-62, 1954.

Miller, J. and Yoder, D.: An ontogenetic language teaching strategy for retarded children. In Schiefelbush, R. L. and Lloyd, L. L. (Eds.): *Language perspectives: Acquisition, retardation and intervention.* Baltimore, Maryland: Univ Park, 1974.

Moores, D. F.: Psycholinguistics and deafness. *Am Ann Deaf, 115:*37-48, 1970.

Morehead, D. M.: The study of linguistically deficient children. In Singh, S. (Ed.): *Measurement procedures in speech, hearing and language.* Baltimore, Maryland: Univ Park, 1975.

Morehead, D. M. and Ingram, D.: The development of base syntax in normal and linguistically deviant children. *J Speech Hear Res, 16:*330-352, 1973.

Morehead, D. M. and Morehead, A. E. (Eds.): *Normal and deficient child language.* Baltimore, Maryland: Univ Park, 1976.

Morris, W. (Ed.): *The American heritage dictionary of the English language.* New York: HM, 1969.

Newfield, M. U. and Schlanger, B. B.: The acquisition of English morphology by normal and educable mentally retarded children. *J Speech Hear Res, 11:*693-706, 1968.

Piaget, J.: *The origins of intelligence in children.* New York: Basic, 1952.

Presnell, L. M.: Hearing-impaired children's comprehension and production of syntax in oral language. *J Speech Hear Res, 16:*12-21, 1973.

Rees, N. S.: Pragmatics of language: Applications to normal and disordered language development. In Schiefelbusch, R. L. (Ed.): *Bases of language intervention*. Baltimore, Maryland: Univ Park, 1978.

Rimland, B.: *Infantile autism*. New York: Appleton-Century-Crofts, 1969.

Rosenthal, W. S.: Perception of temporal order in aphasic and normal children as a function of certain stimulus parameters. Unpublished doctoral dissertation, Stanford University, Stanford, California, 1970.

Ross, L. E. and Leavitt, L. A.: Process research: Its use in prevention and intervention with high risk children. In Tjossem, T. D. (Ed.): *Intervention strategies for high risk infants and young children*. Baltimore, Maryland: Univ Park, 1976.

Schlanger, B.: Speech measurements of institutionalized mentally handicapped children. *Am J Ment Defic, 58*:114-122, 1953a.

Schlanger, B.: Speech examination of a group of institutionalized mentally handicapped children. *J Speech Hear Disord, 18*:339-349, 1953b.

Schlesinger, I. M.: Production of utterances and language acquisition. In Slobin, D. I. (Ed.): *The ontogenesis of grammar*. New York: Acad Pr, 1971.

Schwartz, E. R.: Characteristics of speech and language development in the child with myelomeningocele and hydrocephalus. *J Speech Hear Disord, 39*:465-468, 1974.

Semmel, M. I. and Greenough, D.: Comprehension and imitation of sentences by Down's syndrome children as a function of transformational complexity. *Am J Ment Defic, 75*:739-746, 1971.

Simmons-Martin, A. A.: The oral-aural procedure: Theoretical basis and rationale. *Volta Review, 74*:541-551, 1972.

Shirley, H.: *Pediatric psychiatry*. Cambridge, Massachusetts: Harvard U Pr, 1963.

Slobin, D. I.: *Psycholinguistics*. Glenview, Illinois: Scott F, 1971.

Slobin, D. I.: Cognitive prerequisites for the development of grammar. In Ferguson, C. A. and Slobin, D. I. (Eds.): *Studies of child language development*. New York: HR & W, 1973.

Snyder, L. S.: Pragmatics in language disabled children: Their prelinguistic and early verbal performatives and presuppositions. Unpublished doctoral dissertation, University of Colorado, Boulder, Colorado, 1975.

Sommers, R. K. and Starkey, K. L.: Dichotic verbal processing in Down's syndrome children having qualitatively different speech and language skills. *Am J Ment Defic, 82*:44-53, 1977.

Spreen, O.: Language functions in mental retardation—A review. *Am J Ment Defic, 69*:482-494, 1965.

Stark, J. A.: A comparison of the performance of aphasic children on three sequencing tests. *J Commun Disord, 1*:31-34, 1967.

Stoller, P. (Ed.): *Black American English: Its background and its usage in the schools and in literature*. New York: Dell, 1975.

Tallal, P. and Newcombe, F.: Impairment of auditory perception and language comprehension in dysphasia. *Brain and Language, 5*:13-24, 1978.

Tallal, P. and Piercy, M.: Defects of non-verbal auditory perception in children with developmental aphasia. *Nature (London), 241*:468-469, 1973a.

Tallal, P. and Piercy, M.: Developmental aphasia: Impaired rate of non-verbal processing as a function of sensory modality. *Neuropsychologia, 11*:389-398, 1973b.

Tallal, P. and Piercy, M.: Developmental aphasia: Rate of auditory processing and selective impairment of consonant perception. *Neuropsychologia, 12*:83-93, 1974.

Tallal, P. and Piercy, M.: Developmental aphasia: The perception of brief vowels and extended consonants. *Neuropsychologia, 13*:69-74, 1975.

Tallal, P., Stark, R. E., and Curtiss, B.: Relation between speech perception and speech production impairment in children with developmental dysphasia. *Brain and Language, 3*:305-317, 1976.

Taylor, O. and Swinney, D.: The onset of language. In Irwin, J. V. and Marge, M. (Eds.): *Principles of childhood language disabilities.* New York: Appleton-Century-Crofts, 1972.

Tjossem, T. D.: Early intervention: Issues and approaches. In Tjossem, T. D. (Ed.): *Intervention strategies for high risk infants and young children.* Baltimore, Maryland: Univ Park, 1976.

Tracy, S.: My philosophy of the education of the deaf. *Am Ann Deaf, 107*: 260-268, 1962.

Vernon, M.: Sociological and psychological factors in profound hearing loss. *J Speech Hear Res, 12*:541-563, 1969.

Vygotsky, L. S.: *Thought and language.* Translated by E. Haufmann and G. Vakar. Cambridge, Massachusetts: MIT Pr, 1962.

Weiner, P. S.: The perceptual level functioning of dysphasic children: A follow-up study. *J Speech Hear Res, 15*:423-438, 1972.

Weir, R.: *Language in the crib.* Hague: Mouton, 1962.

Wender, P. H.: *Minimal brain dysfunction in children.* New York: Wiley, 1971.

West, J. J. and Weber, J. L.: A linguistic analysis of the morphemic and syntactic structures of a hard of hearing child. *Language and Speech, 17*: 68-79, 1974.

West, R. (Ed.): *Childhood aphasia. Proceedings of the Institute on Childhood Aphasia.* California Society for Crippled Children and Adults, San Francisco, 1962.

Wheldall, K.: Receptive language development in the mentally handicapped. In Perry, P. (Ed.): *Language and communication in the mentally handicapped.* Baltimore, Maryland: Univ Park, 1976.

Wiig, E.: Language disabilities of adolescents. *Br J Disord Commun, 11*:3-17, 1976.

Wilhelm, H. and Lovaas, O. I.: Stimulus overselectivity: A common feature in autism and mental retardation. *Am J Ment Defic, 81*:19-25, 1976.

Willbrand, M. L.: Language acquisition: The continuing development from nine to ten years. In Ingemann, F. (Ed.): *Mid-America linguistics conference reports.* Lawrence, Kansas: University of Kansas, 1976.

Willbrand, M. L.: Semantic intent and interpretation—beware! *J Tenn Speech Hear Assoc, 22*:21-25, 1977a.

Willbrand, M. L.: Psycholinguistic theory and therapy for initiating two-word utterances. *Br J Disord Commun, 12*:37-46, 1977b.

Williams, F. (Ed.): *Language and poverty: Perspectives on a theme.* Chicago: Markham, 1970.

Williams, R. and Wolfram, W.: Social dialects: Differences *vs.* disorders. American Speech and Hearing Association, Special Project, Report of the Committee on Communication Behavior and Problems in Urban Populations, Rockville, Md. 1977.

Yoder, D. E.: Some viewpoints of the speech, hearing and language clinician. In Williams, F. (Ed.): *Language and poverty.* Chicago: Markham, 1970.

Zangwill, O. L.: The relation of nonverbal cognitive functions to aphasia. In Lenneberg, E. H. and Lenneberg, E. (Eds.): *Foundations of language development,* vol. 2. New York: Acad Pr, 1975.

Zeaman, D. and House, B. J.: The role of attention in retardate discrimination learning. In Ellis, N. R. (Ed.): *Handbook of mental deficiency.* New York: McGraw, 1963.

Chapter 3

FORMAL ASSESSMENT AND EVALUATION
OF LANGUAGE DISORDERS

THE MAIN PURPOSES of formalized language testing are to evaluate how a particular child compares with his peer group in language development and skills and to get as much information about the language skills a child has in his repertoire, as measured by different tests, as possible in a small amount of time. In order to achieve the first purpose and to establish whether the child has significantly disordered language, it is necessary to use norm-referenced tests since such tests will have information on how a larger peer group would perform on the test (standard performance). The second purpose can be met by using a criterion-referenced test that assesses a large number of expected behaviors in each of the various language domains and uses structured elicitations to quickly estimate whether or not the child has in his repertoire the skills necessary for executing or handling the various items in the test.

Following formal testing, it is necessary to observe the child in a "low structured" or informal situation to more nearly identify the specific language problems that the child may be having. The present chapter will be devoted to a discussion of formal testing that might be used to detect the presence of a language disorder. The next chapter will review informal evaluation procedures necessary to identify exactly what specific problems the child is having and what target objectives may need to be set up for treatment.

The two major types of formal testing are norm-referenced testing and domain-referenced testing. Since speech pathologists often find themselves engaged in either constructing tests or evaluating the quality of tests, standards for constructing and evaluating both types of formal tests are presented below. Additionally, specialized testing procedures for assessing language processing disorders are discussed. The last portion of this chapter presents brief descriptions of a number of standardized tests that can be used for language assessment. This list of tests is not meant to be exhaustive, but merely representative of current tests being used.

Norm-referenced versus Domain-referenced Testing

Tests that interpret performance scores in terms of how a person compares to the scores of persons in representative groups are called norm-referenced tests. Much of our test theory and practice is based on norm-referenced testing (Gronlund, 1973). The score of an individual is interpreted in terms of the relative position of that score in the distribution of scores of the norm group. For example, a score of 45 on a particular test might warrant assigning the child to the 80th percentile; this means that only 20 percent of the normative reference group scored higher than this person on the test and that 80 percent of the group scored lower. Interpretation is always made in terms of a person's standing relative to other persons. Another kind of interpretation, which refers mainly to what tasks on the test the person being tested could or could not perform depending upon what the test measures, is called a domain-referenced interpretation. It is possible to arrive at both norm-referenced and domain-referenced interpretations of a standardized test; for example, we could say that a person surpassed 80 percent of the norm group (norm-referenced interpretation) by correctly passing 85 percent of the items on the test (content-referenced interpretation). "The two types of interpretation are likely to be most meaningful, however, when the test is designed specifically for the type of interpretation to be made" (Gronlund, 1977, p. 15).

Norm-referenced Tests

The major steps in constructing a norm-referenced test are (1) development of a set of items that will tap the behaviors to be assessed, ranging from easy to difficult; (2) statement of the items in either general or specific terms; (3) assessment of the items' ability to discriminate "good" scorers from "poor" scorers; (4) assessment of the test's temporal and internal reliability; (5) selection of a norm group that is representative of the population with whom the test will be used (a group whose scores will be distributed widely along the scale); (6) development of some standardized interpretation of the various test scores; and (7) establishment of evidence of various types of validity.

The first step above, development of items, is best achieved by developing a table of specifications that lists content areas along the ordinate and specific behavioral outcomes along the abscissa and then determining the number of items for each cell in the table. A hypothetical table of specifications for a norm-referenced language test is presented in Table I. The numbers in the cells represent the possible number of items that test the behavioral objectives under the various content areas. Items for each cell should represent as wide a range of difficulty as possible. Level of difficulty of each item can be assessed after a preliminary normative sample has been tested. The difficulty of an item is expressed as the percent of the sample passing it.

The second step, defining items, is concerned with providing a broad coverage of behavioral objectives with as few items as possible. Since Table I suggests a total of 136 items for coverage, such a test will probably be unwieldy. Its efficiency may be stepped up by constructing a fair number of broad-based or general items and including only specific items for behaviors that cannot be adequately assessed via items with a broader base.

The third step, assessment of discrimination power of each

TABLE I

SPECIFICATIONS FOR A NON-REFERENCED TEST OF
LANGUAGE DEVELOPMENT

| | Behavioral Objectives | | | | | |
| | Comprehends | | | Produces | | |
Content Areas	Forms	Functions	Uses	Forms	Functions	Uses
Pragmatics		5	5		5	5
Semantics	5	5	5	5	5	.5
Morphology	3	3	3	3	3	3
Basic Syntax	3	3	3	3	3	3
Transformations	5	5	5	5	5	5
Phonology	10			10		

item, is achieved by determining the extent to which each item differentiates good scorers from poor scorers on the total test. A simple method of estimating item discrimination power is to compare the number of the highest scoring 30 percent and the number of the lowest scoring 30 percent who passed the item. This equation is expressed as follows (Gronlund, 1977, p. 112):

$$D = \frac{Ru - Rl}{1/2 \ T}$$

Where D = the index of discriminating power, Ru = the number in the upper group passing the item, Rl = the number in the lower group passing the item, and $\frac{1}{2}T$ = one half of the total number of persons included in the item analysis (i.e. U + L/2). Items that have a discrimination power of 0.50 or above are very desirable; those whose discrimination power is near zero should be eliminated.

The fourth step, assessing reliability, is best achieved by attempting a multiple evaluation approach. The reliability coefficient tells what proportion of the test variance is nonerror variance. It increases as test length increases; it also increases as a function of spread or variance of scores. Table II (from Gronlund, 1977, p. 139) suggests a broad-based program of evaluating reliability.

TABLE II

METHODS OF ESTIMATING RELIABILITY*

Method	Type of Information Provided
Test-retest method	The stability of test scores over some given period of time
Equivalent-forms method	The consistency of the test scores over different forms of the test (i.e., different samples of items)
Test-retest with equivalent forms	The consistency of the test scores over *both* a time interval and different forms of the test
Internal-consistency methods	The consistency of the test scores over different parts of the test.

* Scorer reliability should also be considered when evaluating the responses to supply-type items (e.g. interview tests). This is typically done by having the sample scored independently by two scorers and then correlating the two sets of scores. Agreement among scorers, however, is not a substitute for the methods of estimating reliability shown in the table. From N. E. Gronlund, *Constructing Achievement Tests*, 2nd ed., © 1977, p. 139. Reprinted by permission of Prentice-Hall, Inc., Englewood Cliffs, New Jersey.

A coefficient of stability (test-retest) is obtained by correlating two successive administrations of the test on the same subjects; there is usually an interval of about two to three weeks between testings.

A coefficient of equivalence (alternate forms) can be obtained by constructing two independent forms of the test designed to assess the same content areas and behavioral objectives; a correlation of scores on the two forms administered to the same group, with the order of the forms being randomized, will yield a reliability index.

The test-retest with equivalent forms requires that the different forms of the test be administered after an intervening period of time; this is the most dependable estimate of reliability since it takes into account a great number of sources of score variation (Cronbach, 1970).

The internal consistency of a test is often assessed by correlating the odd items with the even items of the test (split-half method). With developmental tests that utilize a basal and ceiling procedure in administration, the split-half estimate of reliability will be spuriously high since odd and even items below the basal and above the ceiling will automatically be scored the same. We feel that a more appropriate method of estimating internal consistency is to utilize the Kuder-Richardson formula, which assesses consistency of student responses from item to item and yields a more conservative estimate.

Step five above, selecting a norm group, is a very important step in terms of test interpretation since it determines the reference against which the score of any single person will be compared. The score of any person should be compared to the scores of a group having the same age, socioeconomic status, linguistic environment, etc. as the group with whom he is expected to compete. Characteristics of the norm group should be made clearly known in the manual. Age level, for example, should be reported in years and months rather than grade level, since age of any grade will vary depending on the time of year the testing is completed. Although sex is not considered a variable in language evaluation, most sample experts recommend that sex be equally balanced. Also, if one is desirous of comparing a child against a specialized population—such as mentally retarded, cerebral palsied, etc.—standardized information should be made available from a representative sample of each type of disorder.

Step six, standardizing scores for test interpretation, is a most important one because a raw score in and of itself does not mean anything on a norm-referenced test. A raw score of 40 on two different tests does not necessarily represent the same value. In order for scores on two different tests to be compared, they must first be equated through a standardization "transformation." A common transformation is the z-score in which each score on a test is subtracted from the mean score (M) of the standard or norm group and divided by the corresponding standard deviation (S.D.). If on one test M = 30 and S.D. = 4 and on another test M = 50 and S.D. = 6, a z-score for the raw score of 40 on the first test would be

$$\frac{40-30}{4} = 2.5$$

whereas the z-score for the raw score of 40 on the second test would be

$$\frac{40-50}{6} = -1.7$$

Sometimes a T-score is used as the standardized score for any particular raw score; this is the z-score multiplied by 10 and added to an arbitrary mean of 50. A T-score eliminates the negative and decimal values that are encountered in using z-scores. The T-scores for the above raw scores (40 and 40) would be 75 and 33 respectively (one substantially above normal and the other substantially below normal).

Other raw score transformations that are less powerful but that represent equivalent values across different tests are percentiles (a point on a scale of scores at which or below which a given percent of the norm group fell) and stanine scores, with the following percentage of norm group scores falling at each stanine: stanine 1 = 4 percent of the norm group whose scores fell around 2 S.D. below the mean, stanine 2 = 7 percent of the norm group whose scores fell around 1.5 S.D. below the mean, stanine 3 = 12 percent of the norm group whose scores fell around 1 S.D. below the mean, stanine 4 = 17 percent of the norm group whose scores fell around 0.5 S.D. below the mean, stanine 5 = 20 percent of the norm group whose scores fell approximately at the mean, stanine 6 = 17 percent of the norm group whose scores fell around 0.5 S.D. above the mean, stanine 7 = 12 percent of the norm group whose scores fell around 1.5 S.D. above the mean, and stanine 9 = 4 percent of the norm group whose scores fell around 2 S.D. above the mean. Grade-level or age-equivalent scores, which represent age or grade-level at which the majority of the norm group received a particular raw score on the test, are often used but are not highly recommended.

The seventh step in the construction and evaluation of a norm-referenced test (the validation step) is probably the most difficult one. Table III (from Gronlund, 1977, p. 131) shows the most widely agreed upon types of validity and questions that are addressed by each type. In achievement tests such as those used for assessing language, content validity is the primary concern, although the other types of validity are also of some importance; content validity is of great concern in domain-referenced tests (discussed later in this chapter). Collecting evidence of validity requires ongoing research; it cannot be measured, it can only be inferred. It is usually expressed in terms of degree (for example, low, moderate, or high).

Probably the most important component of content validity

TABLE III

BASIC TYPES OF VALIDITY

Type	*Question to Be Answered*
Content validity	How adequately does the test content sample the larger universe of situations it represents
Criterion-related validities	How well does test performance predict future performance (predictive validity) or estimate present standing (concurrent validity) on some other valued measure called a CRITERION?
Construct validity	How well can test performance be explained in terms of psychological attributes?

* From N. E. Gronlund, *Constructing Achievement Tests*, 2nd ed., © 1977, p. 131. Reprinted by permission of Prentice-Hall, Inc., Englewood Cliffs, New Jersey.

is the adequacy of test items in sampling the "universe" of the domain being tested. The table of specification described in step one (see Table I) for constructing a test is the best way to try to increase adequacy of the sample of items to be used. Unfortunately, there is no simple statistical procedure for determining the adequacy of content validity. "Whether a test is constructed or selected, the evaluation of content validity is a rather long, involved process based on careful logical analysis" (Gronlund, 1977, p. 133).

Criterion-related validity includes predictive validity and concurrent validity. The most important indicator of both of these types of validity is the degree of relationship between the test and another criterion to which it logically should relate (such as another established test for concurrent validity or academic achievement for predictive validity). Another indicator of criterion-related validity that can be devised is an expectancy table. This is a two-fold chart with categorical performance on the test down the left side of the chart and categorized performance on the criterion, e.g. reading level, used across the top. Table IV is an example of such an expectancy table. A chi square (X^2) test for K independent samples or a contingency coefficient (Siegel, 1956) can be calculated on the basis of these figures in the table to see the degree to which the distribution of frequencies on the test relates to the distribution of the criterion measure. X^2 for the hypothetical figures in Table IV is significant beyond the 0.001 level of confidence and the contingency coefficient (if N = 100) equals 0.805.

Construct validity is essential to any test that purports to mea-

TABLE IV

EXPECTANCY TABLE SHOWING THE RELATION BETWEEN
READING PLACEMENT LEVEL AND SCORES ON A LANGUAGE TEST
(SIMULATED DATA)

Grouped Language Test Scores (Stanines)	Low	Reading Group Middle	High
Above Average (7, 8, 9)		24	76
Average (4, 5, 6)	5	65	30
Below Average (1, 2, 3)	67	25	8

sure some underlying personality trait or quality; however, it is probably not as essential in language testing as content validity. "The key element in construct validity . . . is the *experimental verification* of the test interpretations we propose to make. This involves a wide variety of procedures and many different types of evidence. As evidence accumulates concerning the meaning of the test scores, our interpretations are enriched and we are able to make them with greater confidence" (Gronlund, 1977, p. 137).

The appendix of this chapter presents a number of standardized language tests that are currently available for use; the presentation gives general identification information, estimated cost, brief description of the purpose and nature of the test, practical aspects, standardization information (including norms and reliability and validity estimates), strengths, and major needs. It is important to remember not to use norm-referenced tests over and over, to insure the child is not being allowed to learn the test.

Domain-referenced Tests

In constructing domain-referenced tests, the tasks are a little different. Instead of choosing a few items to represent a broad range of skills, one needs to keep in mind that this test will be used to test a person's repertoire of knowledge or skills and therefore must contain a much larger number of items in each cell; items in each cell need to serve as a representative sample of a specified domain of skills. The purpose of a domain-referenced test is not to identify where a child stands in comparison to a group, but rather to find out what the child has or has not achieved in a particular behavioral domain area. The level of achievement is usually expressed as a ratio between actual mastery and some predetermined expected level of mastery.

There are several reasons why norm-referenced tests do not serve well as domain-referenced or mastery tests (Gronlund, 1973, p. 3): (1) The "conglomerate" of items usually does not provide an adequate description of a child's achievement repertoire. This is especially true where only a few items represent each area of achievement. (2) Norm-referenced tests automatically omit items that are passed by an entire group, yet these items would be of interest in taking an inventory of what a particular child can do. (3) If the test uses multiple-choice items, e.g. the NSST or TACL, some correct answers could be due to chance and this would distort the accuracy in mapping the achievement repertoire of an individual child.

There are some additional limitations imposed by use of a norm group as a standard (Hersen and Berlow, 1976, p. 15). Collection of a large group of clients "homogeneous for a particular behavior disorder" is often difficult; therefore, what is usually used as a standard is a large group of persons who do not manifest the behavior disorder in question or, if it is present, it is masked by the overwhelming variables of heterogeneity. Variance obtained in normative assessment is intersubject variance, since each subject is tested only once; the practice of generalizing intersubject validity and reliability as representative of intrasubject validity and reliability could be fraught with pitfalls. Use of the domain-referenced test for measuring progress over time through repeated testing makes norm-referencing irrelevant.

Domain-referenced tests can be used for assessing intrasubject variability as well as strengths and weaknesses of a child in various domains by analyzing the proportion of objectives in a domain that the child performs at different points in time. In this sense, they become powerful diagnostic tests for assessing needs as well as progress. A major strength of the domain tests is their ability to provide a more precise basis for planning instructional objectives and for analyzing progress being made in various content domains during the intervention process.

Criterion-referenced domain testing carries mastery testing a step further, in that, in addition to detailed assessment of mastery in somewhat narrowly defined domains, it specifies a specific criterion for estimating degree of mastery in a domain or degree of progress toward an objective. Thus, mastery of the "is verbing" construction might be a particular objective in the language domain, but a criterion reference of percent of time "is verbing" is used correctly by the child would give additional information regarding the degree of progress toward goal mastery.

The general notion of criterion testing, using degree of mastery, followed a wave of interest in programmed instruction patterned after Skinner's teaching machine concept. "The gist of this method is to treat each response as a test that is to be reinforced or not, depending on success" (Donlon, 1975, p. 29).

An example of a domain-referenced test that specifies a large number of objectives to be assessed under various language domains is the *System FORE: Developmental Language Program* (Clark, 1972). Table V gives the specifications for this domain-referenced test. The numbers within the cells represent the number of items or objectives being tested at each level in each domain. Scoring of items is dichotomous, i.e. it is done in terms of mastery or nonmastery.

In a sense, any program of instruction that contains a rather

Table V. Specification table for Los Angeles system, FORE: Developmental Language Program (Clark, 1972).

Domain *Levels**	*Phonology*	*Morphology/Syntax*		*Semantics* *Receptive*	*Expressive*	*Total*
0	7	4		5	6	22
1	3	5		5	4	17
2	6	8		4	5	23
3	7	13		8	6	34
4	8	11		6	8	33
5	6	8		4	6	24
6	10	6		2	6	24
7	7	5	6	9		27
8	9	5	3	8		25
9	5	1	3	6		15
10	5	2	2	6		15
11	10	8	3	7		28
12	8	2	4	10		24
13	9	2	4	12		27
14	7	3	5	8		23
15	8	3	4	2		17
16	4	7	6	6		23
17	8	4	1	2		15
18	10	8	2	7		27
Total	137	50	55 · 43	34	83 · 41	443

*Differing levels of difficulty.

detailed sample of items representative of a larger domain-universe can be used for domain or content testing. Wherever criteria are given in such a program for assessing entry and exit levels or for assessing relative progress toward mastery of objectives, items of the program can be used for criterion-referenced testing. Domain testing enables one to assess presence or absence of item mastery, whereas, criterion testing permits greater precision in testing by determining degree of mastery or nonmastery for particular objectives. Criterion testing allows one to establish what is commonly referred to as a base level. A base level is the child's present degree of mastery of a particular objective and may be designated by different terms such as percent level of mastery for developmental tasks, percent of correct performance in the case of a transitional behavioral-task, or frequency of occurrence of a behavior that is being encouraged. A baseline is the intersect line across several periods of observation; it is a line connecting frequency points or levels of mastery (often the 50 percent level is considered a base level at which intervention should begin).

Criterion testing often uses error-rate rather than frequency of correct performance as a basic measure; this is especially useful when an erroneous or interfering behavior needs to be extinguished. An example of this is using reduction of the *me* substitute for *I* in spontaneous communication as an indication of increased language maturation; in this case it is necessary to establish the base-level frequency of the behavior. The clinician should take at least two spontaneous samples prior to treatment; in the samples a count is made of the number of times the first person pronoun is used incorrectly. Then the clinician tries to reduce this frequency level to zero through the use of various intervention strategies. To determine the point at which the child reaches criterion, one or more samples need to be taken.

The philosophy of domain testing is dedicated to the idea that teaching and learning can be improved if clinicians and teachers operationally specify objectives to be taught and develop criterion-referenced tests to assess student progress toward those objectives. Prerequisite skills for placement in an objectives-curriculum is best assessed by domain-referenced (DR) testing (Gronlund, 1977, p. 19). Also assessment of teachability of objectives can best be approached through DR assessment. A third function of domain-referenced testing is to assess generalizability or transfer of learned skills.

Since criterion or domain tests are not used for comparing students, discrimination power of items is of little value. All students could correctly answer some items on a domain test; thus, such items would have zero discrimination power, yet they would still give information on what students know or can do, and to eliminate such items would distort the true assessment.

The most important concern in evaluating domain-referenced tests "is extent to which each item is measuring the effects of instruction. If an item can be answered correctly by all students both before and after instruction, the item obviously is not measuring instructional effects. Similarly, if an item is answered incorrectly by all students both before and after instruction, the item is not serving its intended function" (Gronlund, 1977, p. 115).

Obtaining a measure of instructional effects is one way of determining item quality. Item sensitivity to instructional outcome can be analyzed by the following formula:

$$S = \frac{RA - RB}{T}$$

Where RA = number of students answering the item correctly after instruction; RB = number of students answering the item correctly before instruction; and T = total number of students answering the item both times (Gronlund, 1977, p. 115).

Sensitivity of an item might be a measure of instructional effectiveness rather than item sensitivity. Also testing effects may influence outcome of test-retest. These must be considered as possible variables; but analysis should still be made since it is the only way to determine sensitivity of items to instruction (Gronlund, 1977, p. 116).

Score interpretation is the area in which domain-referenced tests differ most greatly from norm-referenced tests. Items missed on the domain test are of central importance since they are the ones around which remedial work will center.

The most important type of validity of domain-referenced tests is content validity, since these tests purport to measure what the child can or cannot do. A table of specifications helps in establishing the domains to be tested and learning outcomes that are essential. If the test is constructed to closely fit a good table of specifications, it is more likely to have good content validity.

Concurrent and construct validity can be arrived at in the same way as for norm-referenced tests. Without content validity, however, it is impossible for domain tests to possess predictive, relational, or experimental validity.

It is desirable for domain-referenced tests to be reliable in the same ways that norm-referenced tests are. "Unfortunately, our means for estimating these types of consistency do not match our need for such information. Since criterion-referenced mastery tests are not designed to discriminate among individuals, and thus variability need not be present in the scores, the traditional correlational estimates of reliability are inappropriate" (Gronlund, 1977, p. 123). Domain-referenced tests have one characteristic that helps insure greater reliability; the longer a test, the more reliable it tends to be. Domain-referenced tests are noted for their great number of items.

A word or two of precaution against attempts to "norm-reference" domain-referenced tests. First, it may be undesirable to try to "normalize" all behaviors across various subcultures. Second, normalization may serve to promote uniformity and regimentation rather than diversity due to a tendency for desired behavior to cluster closely around the mean. Third, norm-referencing a domain of behaviors does not necessarily improve or prove a test's validity. A test could have an excellently standardized norm-reference group and still have poor content validity; strict standardization on a large representative group could falsely be interpreted by users to mean that the test has good validity. Also trying to force a domain-referenced test to have high correlational reliability might distort the fidelity of the domain-referenced test, as has previously been mentioned. Norm-referenced tests may have even poorer content validity due to sparsity of items representing each domain and due to elimination of easy items.

Now a word of precaution relative to use of domain-ref-

CHECKLIST

	Yes	No
Adequacy of the Test Plan		
1. Does the test plan include a detailed description of the instructional objectives and the content to be measured?	___	___
2. Does the table of specifications clearly indicate the relative emphasis to be given to each objective and each area of content?	___	___
3. Is the standard of performance reasonable for the learning outcomes to be measured?	___	___
Adequacy of the Test Items		
4. Are the types of test items appropriate for the learning outcomes to be measured?	___	___
5. Do the test items measure an adequate sample of student performance for each type of interpretation to be made?	___	___
6. Do the test items present clear and definite tasks to be performed?	___	___
7. Are the test items free of nonfunctional material?	___	___
8. Are the test items of appropriate difficulty for the learning outcomes to be measured?	___	___
9. Are the test items free of technical defects (clues, ambiguity, inappropriate reading level)?	___	___
10. Is the answer to each test item one that experts would agree upon?	___	___
11. Are the items of each type in harmony with the rules for constructing that item type?	___	___
Adequacy of the Test Format		
12. Are the test items that measure the same instructional objective grouped together in the test?	___	___
13. Are the test items arranged in order of increasing difficulty within each section of the test and within the test as a whole?	___	___

14. Does the item layout on the page contribute to ease of reading and ease of scoring?   —— ——
15. Are the test items numbered in consecutive order?   —— ——
16. Are specific, clear directions provided for each section of the test and for the test as a whole?   —— ——

---

erenced tests. Professional sophistication in development and use of such tests is still in its infancy; it is still a bootstrap type of operation. Use of such tests should probably be restricted to determining entry and exit levels in a curriculum and for planning teaching strategies*; great caution should be used in any attempts to use the tests as predictors of future outcomes or for indirectly assessing inherent traits of an individual in the same sense that norm-referenced tests are used.

The checklist above is suggested by Gronlund (1973, pp. 51-52) for evaluating tests prepared for criterion-referenced use. Positive answers to this list are desirable while negative answers indicate errors in construction that should be corrected before using the test.

Testing Verbal Information Processing Skills

In Chapter 1 various processing functions were described as probably playing an important role in language; and in Chapter 2 we described processing problems relating to attention, recognition memory, memory for sequences, semantic memory, and motor production that were frequently found associated with language disorders. The present chapter will discuss briefly some resources that can be used to assess these various verbal-information processing skills.

---

* Discrimination must be used in employing test items as curriculum targets. There may be a danger of using the same objectives and activities for all children, at the expense of individual programming. Also, it may be possible to teach fragmented tasks independent of the general growth of the individual or apart from the contextual situation where tasks are normally used; for example, a child may learn to discriminate sizes and shapes on geometrical form boards and not be able to generalize these skills to objects encountered in functional life activities (Stillman, 1974).

Attention

An instrument for screening selective auditory attentional deficits in infants was developed and standardized on 480 infants in Sweden by Junker (1972). This test, called the *BEOL* (acronym for the Swedish title), was designed primarily to be used with infants under one year of age. It may prove to be useful with young handicapped children who are relatively free of hearing or motor handicaps. Test-retest reliability estimates on 69 infants indicated the following reliabilities: motor stability test = 0.86; eye contact test = 0.87; attention, visual/tactile = 0.87; attention, visual = 0.79; and attention, auditory = 0.85. One major problem with this test is that the item instructions are not as explicit as one would like to see. A child who responds positively to most of the items on this test should be capable of attending well enough to respond to verbal training.

Another standardized instrument that was not designed specifically for attentional assessment but that contains subtests that can be reliably given to assess visual attention is the *Ordinal Scale of Psychological Development* by Uzgiris and Hunt (1975). As Uzgiris and Hunt suggest, "One need not make use of all the scales. While for many purposes it may be desirable to present all of the situations constituting a particular scale, it is perfectly sensible (given the ordinal nature of these scales) to use specified steps in particular scales to investigate the effects of given kinds of circumstances on development" (p. 145). Any child beyond one year of age should successfully respond to the following subtests on these scales extracted from Uzgiris and Hunt (1975)— if he fails any of them, one may suspect some possible deficits in attentive behaviors.

Detailed descriptions of procedures and materials are given in a book entitled *Assessment in Infancy* (Uzgiris and Hunt, 1975). Materials must be collected by the examiner.

Although this test does not have normative data, its reliability and the high degree of ordinal consistency (OC) of items in each subtest (OC range = 80-99 based on over eighty subjects) enhances its quality as a developmental test.

The *Goldman-Fristoe-Woodcock Auditory Selective Attention*

Items			Test-Retest Reliability	Inter-Observer Agreement (Percent)
I:	1.	Visually follows a slowly moving object.	0.93	100
I:	2.	Notices the disappearance of a slowly moving object.	0.86	91
I:	3.	Finds an object that is partially covered.	0.94	98.6
II:	1.	Displays hand-watching behavior.	0.73	86.7
II:	2.	Visually directs own grasp of object.	0.94	97
II:	4.	Lets go of an object in order to reach for another.	0.47	96
V:	1.	Observes two objects alternately.	0.80	93
V:	2.	Localizes an object by its sound.	0.90	97
V:	4.	Follows the trajectory of a rapidly moving object.	0.92	98
V:	9.	Watches to see where dropped objects land.	0.86	99

Test (a subtest of the *Auditory Skills Test Battery**) purports to assess the ability to attend under increasingly difficult listening conditions. Split-half reliability estimate for this subtest was 0.89. Preliminary validation evidence appears encouraging.

Auditory Memory

RECOGNITION MEMORY. There are very few reliable tests that measure recognition ability independent of comprehension and/ or discrimination. One of the memory tests on the *Goldman-Fristoe-Woodcock Auditory Skills Test Battery*† was designed to

---

* This battery was standardized on over 7,000 subjects from widely differing parts of the United States.

† American Guidance Service, Publisher's Building, Circle Pines, Minnesota 55014.

measure ability to recognize an auditory event that has occurred in the immediate past. The reliability of this subtest was 0.92. This test consists of 110 words divided into five lists of 22 words each recorded on tape. Each word occurs twice within the word list with varying positional locations. The child listens to each word and indicates *yes* or *no* depending on if it has occurred previously in the list.

The *Porch Index of Communication Ability in Children* (Porch, 1974) has some subtests that assess gross recognition ability (perception), but reliability data are not yet available on this test battery. Until such data are available, this test should be used with great caution. Also, its sensitivity to mild or moderate deviations in recognition processing is questionable.

Reaction times in simple recognition tasks may be a sensitive indicator of the recognition process (Sternberg, 1969). Reaction times for recognition average around 0.2 seconds. Aphasic children and adults normally have a slower reaction time, and the magnitude of this latency may be a measure of recognition ability (Warren et al., 1977).

MEMORY FOR SEQUENCING. The *WISC Comprehension* subtest, which measures digit-memory span, has separate standardization data and is acceptably reliable as a test for memory for sequencing. The auditory-sequential-memory subtest on the *ITPA* has been standardized as a subtest and has fairly good reliability. The memory-for-sequence test of the *GFW Auditory Skills Test Battery* is a sequential memory test that does not require a verbal response from the child. The child listens to a prerecorded word list while facing a blank page on the easel-kit. Picture cards are then presented to the child whose task it is to put them in the same segmental order as they occurred on the audiotape. Reliability for this test for the entire normative sample was 0.92. No reliabilities are given for various age levels. The Stanford-Binet digit-memory items may be used to roughly screen memory for sequencing; however, these items do not constitute a subtest on the Stanford-Binet and scores cannot be interpreted separately from the total test score.

SEMANTIC MEMORY. Semantic memory was dichotomized by Guilford (1967) as utilizing two types of information retrieval:

convergent information, in which only a highly specific bit of information can be considered as an appropriate response (an example of such a retrieval is the response expected when a person is asked, "What is your name?"), and divergent information, in which a large variety of retrieved responses could serve equally well and which is dependent upon flexibility of semantic thought (an example of this type of retrieval is when a subject tells about things he or she likes).

Most vocabulary tests, such as the *PPVT* or *Vocabulary Comprehension Scale*, assess to a certain extent long-term semantic memory. Short-term semantic memory can be assessed by use of the *Memory for Content Test* of the *CFW Auditory Skills Test Battery*. In this test, the examiner presents word lists and then shows the child a card containing pictures of all words named plus two that were not named on the list. The child is requested to point to the two pictures that were not named. The reliability of this test for the normative group was 0.86 and for a clinical group was 0.95.

SUMMARY

In review, we have discussed the use of formal testing as a prerequisite to more informal testing to determine whether a particular child has a language problem. We have indicated that norm-referenced tests should be used for comparing a given person to a group of persons. Domain-referenced testing, whose main purpose is to determine what a child has achieved in a domain, is a newer approach to diagnosis and assessment of progress. Construction and validation requisites for formal tests were described.

The following section contains brief summaries of a number of standardized tests. Clinicians must use discretion in choosing appropriate tests to fit the needs for each child or clinical situation. The summaries provided are intended to be informational and not critical reviews; for critical reviews, the reader may wish to refer to Buros (1972) or Darley et al. (in press).

SUMMARIES OF SELECTED
STANDARDIZED TESTS

Assessment of Childen's Language Comprehension

Authors: R. Foster, J. Giddan, and J. Stark.

Publisher, date of publication: Consulting Psychologists Press, 577 College Ave., Palo Alto, California 94306; 1972.

Time required to administer: 10-15 minutes.

Cost: $13.50 (1977).

General type of test: Individual and group forms.

Population for which designed: 3 to 6.11 year old children.

Exact domains being tested: Vocabulary comprehension; comprehension of two, three, and four element sentences.

Subtests and separate scores: Subtest A tests for vocabulary; subtest B tests for comprehension of two critical elements; subtest C tests for comprehension of three critical elements; and subtest D tests for comprehension of four critical elements. The subtests contain fifty, ten, ten, and ten items respectively.

Qualitative features: Picture plates and response forms. A child points to one of a multiple of pictures on each plate.

Scoring procedures: One point for each correct item.

Examiner qualifications and training desired: None specified.

Norms: Mean percentage scores are given for males and females at various ages for each subtest. Percentage is computed by dividing raw score by total possible score on each subtest.

Standardization sample: The normative group consisted of 311 nursery and elementary school children from age 3.0 through 6.9 years. 85 percent of the children were from Florida and 15 percent were from Vermont (Head Start program). 35 percent were from low SES backgrounds and the rest were from low-middle and high-middle SES backgrounds.

Reliability: Split-half (odd versus even items) correlation coefficient of 0.86 was obtained for subtest A and a split-half correlation coefficient of 0.80 was obtained for subtests B, C, and D combined. Number of subjects for these correlations was not reported.

Validity: No validity studies reported.

Major strengths: Can be administered conveniently and rapidly, and requires merely a pointing response on the part of the child. Should serve well as a rapid screening test for auditory comprehension of language in young children.

Major needs: Validity information needs to be reported; also reliability for each of the subtests are not given except for subtest A, which has fifty items. Reliability of subtests B, C, and D could be suspect since they are each comprised of only ten items.

Bankson Language Screening Test*

Author: Nicholas W. Bankson.

Publisher, date of publication: University Park Press, 233 East Redwood Street, Baltimore, Maryland 21202; 1977.

Time required to administer: 25 minutes.

Cost: $14.95 for test; $5.00 for twenty-five answer booklets (1977).

General type of test: Individual screening measure.

Population for which designed: Children ages 4-7; can be used with age 3, but no norms for that age.

Exact domains being tested: (1) Semantic knowledge, (2) morphological rules, (3) syntactical rules, (4) perception, and (5) auditory and visual perception.

Subtests and separate scores: 17 subtests, divided among the five areas tested.

Qualitative features of test materials: Spiral-bound test, colored testing stimuli, self-contained in booklet form.

Scoring procedures: Right-wrong scoring; data can be organized on a profile sheet.

Examiner qualifications and training desired: (1) Examiner should be a professional person for interpretation purposes; (2) Examiner should read test booklet and practice administration five times.

Norms: Based on N of over 600.

Type: Percentile values for children ages 4-8. Mean and standard deviation for each subtest.

Standardization sample: 637 children ages 4.1 to 8.0 from semirural Maryland counties adjacent to the Washington, D.C. metropolitan area. 80 percent were white, 18 percent black, and 2 percent from other nationality groups. The sample came from two preschool classes, nineteen public school classes, and two parochial school classes. Sample ranged from lower-middle to upper-middle class, with 75 percent from a strictly middle-class population.

Reliability: Test-retest, point to point for 70 Ss = 0.94. Kuder-Richardson 20 = 0.96.

Validity: Concurrent; content reported in manual.

Specific procedures followed in assessing validity and results obtained: Correlation of BLST scores with those obtained on PPVT (r = 0.54), Boehm Concept Test (r = 0.62), Test of Auditory Comprehension of Language (r = 0.64). Selected subtests were also compared to performance measured by DSS scoring (r = 0.76) and the Boehm (r = 0.82).

Major strengths: Practicality, simplicity, ease of administration, good correlation with other language measures. Compact, covers a variety of areas.

Major needs: (1) Does not cover pragmatic aspects of language, (2) could benefit from norms at the three-year-old level, since children peak on the

* Information supplied by test's author.

test at the upper age levels, (3) auditory and visual perception subtest not as complete as the morphology, syntax, and semantic subtests, (4) no estimates of reliability for subtest scores are given.

Boehm Test of Basic Concepts*

Author: Ann E. Boehm

Publisher: The Psychological Corporation, 304 East 45th Street, New York, N.Y. 10017.

Date: 1971 edition.

Cost: About $8.50 (1978).

General type of test: Group (at prekindergarten individual administration is recommended; pointing is used as response at prekindergarten instead of marking.)

Population for which designed: Kindergarten, grade one, grade two.

Domains being tested: Designed to measure children's concepts considered necessary for achievement in the first years of school. Specifically covers directions and terms that occur in classrooms and textbooks with considerable frequency and are seldom defined, and relatively abstract basic concepts or ideas found in early curriculum materials, readers, arithmetic, and science books.

Specific concepts: Space, quantity, time, and miscellaneous concepts of different, other, matches, and alike. Heavy emphasis on space (top, farthest, side, etc.) and quantity (some, not many, almost, medium-sized, etc.).

Qualitative features: (a) Pencil and paper, (b) black and white line drawings, (c) four units per page, (d) two test booklets of twenty-five items each for a total of fifty tested items. Second book repeats same concepts as book one, but they are harder to interpret.

Scoring procedures:

  a. Class record form, key, and interpretative aid (in manual)

  b. Class record form grid gives the following:

    1. Total number of children answering correctly

    2. Percent passing each item

    3. Each child's total score on individual items

    4. Percent passing

    5. Percentile for each child

  c. Items are marked with /✔/ if passed correctly.

  d. If items are failed, slot is left blank.

  e. Normative data for each item at kindergarten, grade one, and grade two are given for each test item in the manual.

  f. Detailed directions are given for each test item in the manual.

    1. Key phrases for each item are read twice.

    2. Emphasis is placed on italicized word.

  g. Children may correct errors.

  h. Teacher may assist by indicating appropriate picture set.

Testing time: 15 to 20 minutes.

Examiner qualifications and training desired: None stated specifically al-

---

* Information supplied by Jane M. Carpenter.

though manual talks about "teacher administering test with aids or proctors assisting."

Norms:

a. Population defined and described: Children enrolled in kindergarten, first grade, and second grades in sixteen cities located across the United States were selected. School officials in each cooperating city were asked to provide classroom groups from schools with a fairly wide range of socioeconomic background. For beginning of year testing, 3,517 children were evaluated at kindergarten level, 4,659 children evaluated at first-grade level, and 1,561 children evaluated at second-grade level. For midyear testing, 865 kindergarten children, 991 first-grade children and 813 second-grade children were tested. The children at each level were broken down into low, middle, and high socioeconomic levels. (Specifics on what constitutes definition of socioeconomic level are not given.)

b. Equivalence of Forms A and B. Approximately half of the children at each socioeconomic level in each grade were administered Form A first, followed by Form B given on a different day but within the same week. The other half of the children were tested at the same time but with the forms reversed. Results revealed mean scores on Form A were 42.4 and Form B 42.9. The standard deviations of these scores were 7.3 and 7.0.

c. Tables 5, 6, 7, 8 give the percent of children passing each individual item on the BTBC for both the beginning-of-year standardization sample (separately by grade and socioeconomic level) and middle-of-year standardization. For both from A and B.

The difficulty values given in the norm tables for Form A were entered into the regression equations to obtain estimates of Form B norms for the original standardization sample.

d. Tables 9 and 10 give percentile equivalents of raw scores, by grade and socioeconomic level, for children tested at the beginning and middle of the year.

Data analysis:

a. Percentile equivalents of BTBC total raw scores are given.

b. Means and standard deviations based on the scores obtained are given beneath the percentiles.

c. Interpretative scores are given in the percentile equivalent tables of the raw scores (based on grade level and income).

Reliability:

a. Split-half reliability coefficients for the total score on Form A range from 0.68 to 0.90.

b. Split-half reliability coefficients for the total score on Form B range from 0.12 to 0.94.

(0.12 was obtained for grade 2, high-socioeconomic level sample, which had a mean total score of 48.5 and a standard deviation of 0.9. At this level the value of the BTBC would seem to lie only in the identification of those who are far below the group's average ability.)

c. Standard errors of measurement obtained for BTBC total scores are essentially comparable for Forms A and B.

d. Alternate form reliability coefficients, computed for the total group of students at each of the three grade levels, ranged from 0.55 to 0.92 with a median of 0.76. They tended to be slightly lower in magnitude than those obtained by the split-half method.

Validity: Content validity: The test items were selected from relevant curriculum materials and represent concepts basic to understanding directions and other oral communications from teachers.

Major strengths: Normative data based on large numbers; standarization and reliability statistics.

Major needs: Validity: Construct and concurrent.

Other comments:

1. Suggestions for use of the results in remediation are given in the manual.

2. The BTBC was designed as a screen and teaching instrument rather than for predictive or administrative purposes.

Carrow Elicited Language Inventory*

Author: Elizabeth Carrow.

Publisher: Learning Concepts, 2501 North Lamar, Austin, Texas 78705.

Publishing date: 1974 Edition.

Cost: Kit $49.95 (1977), additional scoring/analysis forms (pkg. 50) $9.50, additional verb protocol sheets (pkg. 50) $9.50.

General type of test: The CELI is a diagnostic test designed for individual administration.

Population for which designed: Children ages 3 through 7.11. The author cautions that the test may not be useful for children who have severe articulation problems that interfere with intelligibility, severe jargon speech, or severe echolalia.

Domains being tested: In the words of the author, this test evaluates the child's "productive control of grammar," involving basic sentence construction types and specific grammatical morphemes. Construction types include forty-seven active sentences and four passives, which in turn are divided into thirty-seven affirmatives and fourteen negatives. The fifty-one stimulus sentences are also classed declarative (37), interrogative (12), and imperative (2). Grammatical categories and features evaluated include articles, adjectives, nouns, noun plurals, verbs, negation, contractions, adverbs, prepositions, demonstratives, and conjunctions. Verbs are evaluated in depth because of the amount of information obtainable from their usage.

Design: Based upon repetition of sentences task, stimuli range in length from two to ten words.

Qualitative features: Tape recorder (not provided), pencil and score sheet, instructions for administration (included in manual), norms and other test development information.

Scoring procedures: Child's performance is transcribed from tape to score sheet.

Marking of errors:
  A. Errors should be marked on the scoring/analysis form in the manner described in the manual (the manual goes into detail on this process, which will not be elaborated here).
  B. Total number of errors per sentence is recorded.
  C. After entire test is scored, the number of errors in each grammatical category (article, noun, etc.) as well as the various types of errors (omission, substitution, etc.) are totaled.
  D. The manual provides special elaboration on what should be considered as a substitution, an omission, etc., as well as how to handle jargon and misarticulations.

Special analysis of verb errors: Provides information about specific types of errors and where they occur.

---

* Information provided by Martin Fujiki.

Testing time: 5 minutes to administer, 20 to 30 minutes to score. (These figures are provided in the Learning Concepts Sales Catalog.)

Examiner qualifications: According to the author, this test was "developed primarily for use by speech pathologists" but "any trained examiner with a background in psycholinguistics and language disorders" may administer and score the test.

Normative population defined and described: 475 white children between the ages of 3.0 and 7.11, in 1973, from middle SES homes in Houston, Texas. Standard American English was the only language spoken in the homes. Children were obtained from day-care centers and church schools. The examiner (who was a speech pathologist) as well as the teacher eliminated any children from the sample with a language or speech disorder. All children were tested by the same examiner using the same instructions.

Type of scores:

A. Percentile ranks with stanine scale corresponding to total raw score.

B. Percentile ranks corresponding to grammar error scores.

C. Percentile ranks corresponding to type of error scores.

Test-retest reliability: Twenty-five children (five at each age 3 through 7) were selected randomly, tested, and retested after a two-week period. The examiner administered, transcribed, and scored both testings. The product-moment correlation coefficient obtained was 0.98.

Interexaminer reliability: Two examiners transcribed and scored ten randomly selected tapes. The coefficient of correlation was 0.98.

Two examiners administered, transcribed, and scored the CELI on twenty children, ten of whom were diagnosed as language disordered. The coefficient of correlation was 0.99.

Validity: Author used statistical methods to show that there was a significant difference in performance from age group to age group, indicating that the scores do improve with age and follow a developmental pattern.

The product-moment correlation coefficient between age and total error score was −0.62.

Another measure of validity was the manner in which the instrument can correctly classify individuals who differ with respect to the variable being measured. Cornelius (1974) tested the ability of the CELI to separate language disordered children from normal children. It was found that the CELI was able to separate these children ($P =$ less than 0.001).

Major strengths: The manual is clear, providing detailed information on all important aspects of the test, as we are cautioning against misuse in many areas.

Major weaknesses: The test may be difficult to score initially, although this is a problem that should be minimized with repeated usage.

Children's Language Processes Inventory*

Author: Barbara B. Hutchinson, Ph.D.

Publisher, date of publication: Conlyn, Inc., P.O. Box 3454, Bloomington, Illinois 61701; 1977.

Time required to administer: Approximately one hour.

Cost: $85.00 (1977).

General type of test: Individual assessment of children's linguistic processes, especially in dysphasia.

Population for which designed: Ages 3 through 12 years.

Exact domains being tested: Dysphasia, MR, visual and visual-motor impairments, language disability.

Subtests and separate scores: Cognitive, auditory, speech, visual-reading, visual-motor-writing. In addition to the five aspects of language tested, mentioned above, there is a rating scale profile chart for other aspects that cannot readily be scored right/wrong.

Qualitative features of test materials: Test kit provides toys for the younger children.

Scoring procedures: Given explicit description in the manual. Number wrong.

Examiner qualifications and training desired: Certified speech pathologist, psychologist, or learning specialist.

Norms: When sufficient data are collected, standard scores and percentiles will be computed for each age. Mean scores with their standard deviations and errors are included in the 1977 edition. Mean rating scale profiles for various groups of children are included in the manual as they apply to the present edition.

Standardization sample: Region: central Illinois. Ages: 3 through 12. Sex: M and F balanced. Subjects obtained from the schools and clinics of this area included 200 normal children and 100 language-impaired. Of the latter, 45 were diagnosed dysphasic, 8 were MR, 19 were language-impaired without the previous two handicaps, 3 were visually impaired without language involvement.

Reliability: Test-retest reliability of the 1977 edition varies according to the subtest from 0.65 to 0.91.

Scorer reliability: 0.96 to 0.99 (two judges, twenty Ss).

Validity: Concurrent validity—0.95 in one instance; 100 percent in another. Thirteen graduate students who were learning to administer the CLPI were judges; subjects were twenty children (including normals) diagnosed by psychologists, teachers, speech pathologists, etc. Students did not know diagnosis of any child. Students gave first and second diagnostic classification to each child tested. Agreement between actual diagnosis and the students' CLPI diagnosis was 95 percent for the first classification; 100 percent for the second.

---

* Information supplied by test's author.

Major strengths: Analyzes children's language difficulties into areas of specific weakness.

Needs: Further validation studies would be helpful.

Developmental Sentence Analysis*

Author: Laura L. Lee.

Publisher: Northwestern University Press, Evanston, Illinois; 1974.

Time for administration: Developmental Sentence Analysis is not a test but is a procedure for analyzing a child's use of grammatical structure from a tape-recorded sample of spontaneous speech in conversation with an adult. The collection of 100 different utterances from the child may take only 15 minutes under normal circumstances, but may take 45-60 minutes from a language-impaired child. The transcription from the tape may take as long as an hour. The classification and scoring of utterances may take another hour. Clearly, this is a procedure that is time-consuming but that may yield extensive information on grammatical development.

Cost: This test is in book form and costs $13.50 (1977).

Purpose and nature of the procedure: It is individually administered by a trained clinician. It is comprised of two parts: (1) developmental sentence types and (2) developmental sentence scoring.

1. Developmental sentence types (DST) is a procedure for classifying the presentence utterances that do not meet the subject-verb requirements of complete sentences. This classification includes noun phrases, locaing and describing utterances, verb phrases, and fragments. Single-word, two-word, and multiword presentences are classified separately, showing increased utterance length. Grammatical development of plurals, verb forms, pronouns, etc. are noted. Thus, a child who does not yet speak in sentences can be shown to have the "building blocks" for further grammatical development.

2. Developmental sentence scoring (DSS) is a procedure for quantifying the development of eight grammatical structures within complete subject-verb sentences: indefinite pronouns, personal pronouns, main verbs, secondary verbs, negatives, conjunctions, interrogatives, and wh- questions. Weighted scores are given for the developmental sequence of grammatical forms within each category. The mean score per sentence is the child's DSS and represents the "grammatical load" that his spontaneous sentences customarily carry. Norms provide comparison of a child's DSS with normally developing children of his chronological age and internal investigation of each category reveals a child's strengths and weaknesses in grammatical development.

The above two procedures allow the analysis of children's grammatical development from early two-word combinations through the use of most adult forms. With this procedure, a clinician can, according to the test's author, evaluate a child's level of grammatical usage in spontaneous speech and can chart his progress in clinical training by comparing successive language samples.

---

* Information supplied by test's author.

Practical aspects: This is a lengthy procedure, not suitable for routine use with all clinical cases. It may be used for setting up training goals and marking progress, especially when a prolonged training period is expected. Clinicians who use this procedure should have considerable background information of grammatical structure. The book includes chapters on basic grammatical structure, instructions for taking a language sample, and detailed information on classifying and scoring utterances.

Standardization information: Norms are based on 200 children, ages 2.0 to 6.11, from middle-income families where standard English was spoken. Norms are presented in tables for developmental sentence types (DST) and in chart form for developmental sentence scoring (DSS). Selected percentiles (10th, 25th, 50th, 75th, and 90th) allow a clinician to estimate a child's percentile for his chronological age group. A clinical child's rate of progress can be compared with that of normally developing children in successive language samples. The book gives extensive discussion of norms and many illustrative language samples are reproduced and analyzed.

Validity and reliability: Extensive statistical information on developmental sentence scoring is provided in a chapter by Roy A. Koenigsknecht and is briefly summarized as follows:

1. The weighted scores for each grammatical structure were determined by a reciprocal averaging procedure that took into account the age at which structures emerged, the consistency of usage, the item-total correlations, and the discrimination of structures between successive age groups.

2. The validity of the DSS was indicated by the significant differences produced between age groups by the over-all scoring procedure and by each of its component grammatical categories.

3. The over-all internal consistency of the DSS as measured by coefficient alpha was 0.71. The within-subject internal consistency was assessed by a split-half procedure in which odd items and even items were combined and then correlated. This resulted in an over-all estimate of reliability of 0.73. Each of the individual grammatical categories was positively correlated with the over-all DSS scores.

4. The stability of the DSS was clearly evidenced by the results of studies of stimulus material differences, temporal reliability, sentence sequence effects, and interviewing clinician differences.

   a. Repeated applications of the DSS indicated that the procedure can be used with different stimulus materials, within the interest range of the child, with consistent overall results.

   b. Although biases do occur when presentations are within short time periods, when repeated measurements are taken over longer time intervals of either four or eight months, increases in the over-all measures are consistent with the developmental pattern suggested from the cross-sectional research.

    c. The effects of warm-up and general adjustment to the conversational setting did not favor significantly better grammatical usage in the later utterances in a corpus.

    d. There was consistency on the DSS samples elicited by different interviewers across three age levels.

Major strengths: Developmental Sentence Analysis provides a clinician with detailed information about a child's use of grammatical structure in spontaneous speech. It allows for effective, individualized lesson planning. Progress in grammatical development can be determined by successive language samples, and a child's increased consistency of usage of individual grammatical forms can be demonstrated.

One rather special application may be for establishing the clinician's accountability for teaching effectiveness. More consistent use of pronouns, more highly developed verb forms, greater use of conjunctions, and other significant increases in grammatical competence can be quantified through pretreatment and posttreatment application of DSA. The over-all mean score per sentence (DSS) can reflect progress being made by rate of development in an individual child. The DSA can be administered as often as desired without invalidating the procedure.

Major needs: Developmental Sentence Analysis requires considerable knowledge of grammatical structure on the part of the clinician. It is a time-consuming procedure that should be used periodically with long-term clinical cases. Content and concurrent validity information would be helpful in evaluating the quality of the procedure.

Hannah-Gardner Preschool Language Screening Test*

Authors: Elaine P. Hannah and Julie Gardner.

Publisher: Joyce Publications, Northridge, California.

Publication date: 1974 edition (out of print).

Description of purpose and nature of test: The Hannah-Gardner is a screening test for preschool children. While not specifically stated, it is assumed that the test administration is to be individual.

Population for which designed: Children ages 3 through 5.5.

Domains tested: Test items are classified as primarily auditory, visual, motor, or conceptual. Auditory and visual tasks are further categorized as primarily memory span, figure-ground, closure, or sequencing tasks. Specific temporal and spatial test items are included on the auditory and motor scales, and a brief linguistic comprehension unit is built into the auditory figure ground section of the auditory scale.

Author's statement: "The present test format taps basic functioning of the auditory, visual, and motor channels, and includes a brief measure of conceptual development."

Subtest and separate scores: Subtests include (1) toddler screening section, (2) visual perception, (3) motor development, (4) auditory perception, (5) conceptual development.

Toddler screening section: Eleven of the test items were answered correctly by all tested subjects in the 3 to 3.5 age group. These items are presented in this section and are directed at children 2.5 to 3 years of age. While no specific standardized scores have been developed for this subtest, the authors' state, ". . . evidence suggests that if children in this age group find these tasks difficult, they should be suspected of being in a high-risk group as far as language development is concerned."

Visual perception subtest: Items are ordered as follows—memory items, figure-ground, closure, and sequencing.

Motor development: Items are ordered as follows—manipulation of objects, copying, hand-finger coordination, skipping, and drawing geometric shapes. (This is a general characterization of the item ordering.)

Auditory perception: Items are ordered as follows—memory, figure-ground linguistic, and figure-ground integration, closure, sequencing, and sound blending.

Conceptual development: Items are ordered as follows—numbers (i.e. give me two blocks), prepositions (put the block in the box), colors, and judgment (show me empty).

A percentile score is obtained on each of these four subtests.

Practical aspects: (1) Materials: test box, three-ring binder, white Styrofoam® ball, red rubber ball, beans, small keg, large keg, various colored

---

* Information supplied by Martin Fujiki.

blocks, spoon, pencil, cup, matchbox, button with buttonhole, orange ball, puzzle, orange square puzzle, eight sets of various cards, six individual cards, picture file (eleven pages), copy-me file (6 pages), test pages (six pages), and test sheets (ten).

(2) Scoring: Each item is scored either 1 or 0. The scores are totaled at the end of each subtest. 10 to 15 seconds are allowed for a response, although additional time may be allowed for the motor activities. The test is not timed, however, the authors feel that administration is smoother if the items are given with little pause between items. The test may be given in two parts, thus allowing for a rest period.

Score interpretation: Subjects falling below the 20th percentile (one standard deviation below the mean) are considered to have a deficit, with from the 20th to the 10th percentile being a gray area, and below the 10th being a definite indication of a deficit. The test is weighted heavily in the auditory and conceptual sections, and thus poor performance in either of these areas will have a strong influence upon the total score (as will good performance).

Testing time: 25 to 35 minutes, depending upon the child's age.

Examiner qualifications: The authors state, "it . . . require(s) little expertise beyond some ability to follow simple directions" to administer this test.

Standardization information: Collection of data: Preliminary normative data were collected from two socioeconomic groups (middle and lower) totalling 180 subjects between the ages of 3 and 5.5 years. Within each age level (3, 3.5, 4, 4.5, 5, 5.5) approximately 14 girls and 16 boys were tested. 90 children were tested in a white, middle-class nursery/kindergarten and 90 children were tested from a Head Start program. All children tested lived in the San Fernando Valley area of Los Angeles. Collection was performed by students enrolled in evaluation classes at California State University, Northridge.

The test norms were originally meant for use by the CSUN Language, Speech, and Hearing Center as area norms. It is recommended by the authors that other centers develop their own normative data for their particular areas.

Reliability: Test-retest reliability: in a preliminary study, twenty randomly selected preschool subjects were tested on two different occasions. (The interval ranged from at least fourteen and not more than twenty-one days.)

The same version was used for each administration. Comparison of the two sets of scores by means of a Pearson Product Moment Statistical Procedure indicated a test-retest reliability correlation of 0.95 between the two administrations. Intratester reliability was 0.93.

Validity: (1) Validity was established by correlation with the ITPA. On a study using twelve children with diagnosed language deficits the following correlations were obtained:

Total Score	0.87†
Auditory Scores	0.55*
Linguistic Comp. (grammatic closure)	0.66*
Linguistic Comp. (grammatic closure)	0.66*
Visual Scores	0.74†
Conceptual Scores (representational subtests)	0.70†

(2) A second study examined whether or not the test could differentiate between subjects with language delay and articulatory deficit. Three groups were used (normal, language delay, and articulatory deficit) with ten subjects in each. A Friedmann Two Way Analysis of Variance technique was used with the following results:

Comparison	*Score*
Total	10.80†
Auditory Score	6.20*
Motor Score	7.80*
Visual Score	11.25†
Conceptual Score	18.20†

Major strengths: Test materials are designed to be of interest to the child. Test takes into account some of the problems in testing young children (short attention span, delayed linguistic development, etc.) and reflects this in scoring.

Major needs or weaknesses: Test needs more extensive normative data. No comment in terms of basal and ceiling scores.

Other comments: This test can be highly useful when used appropriately and within the limits that it was designed for.

---

* Sign at 0.05.
† Sign at 0.01.

The Houston Test of Language Development

Author: Margaret Crabtree.

Publisher, date of publication: Houston Test Co., P.O. Box 35152, Houston, Texas 77035; 1963.

Time required to administer: 30 minutes.

Cost: $27.00 (1974).

General type of test: Individual.

Population for which designed: Part I: 6 to 36 months; part II: 3 to 6 years.

Exact domains being tested: Speech sounds, sentence length and complexity, naming, sensory-motor skills, parts of speech.

Qualitative features of test materials: Kit contains manual, objects and toys, and scoring forms.

Scoring procedures: Binary, correct or incorrect for each item. Raw score is total correct.

Examiner qualifications and training desired: No special preparation specified.

Norms: Age-score equivalents.

Standardization sample: Part II: 102 white children between the ages of 3 and 6 years residing in Houston.

Reliability: No information provided.

Validity: Scores reportedly increase with increasing age.

Major strengths: Developmental test; gives generalized developmental picture of language.

Major needs: Normative data need to be expanded and reliability and validity assessments need to be established.

Language Sampling, Analysis and Training: A Handbook for Teachers and Clinicians*

Authors: Dorothy Tyack and Robert Gottsleben.

Publisher, date of publication: Consulting Psychologists Press, 577 College Ave., Palo Alto, California 94306; 1974.

Time required to administer: 20 minutes (2 to 4 hours to analyze).

Cost: Book and one set of forms about $5.00 (1977).

General type of test: Individual.

Population for which designed: Children with language problems of any age.

Exact domains being tested: Acquisition of syntactic rules. Defines an individual's baseline syntactic skills as well as specific syntactic goals.

Qualitative features of test materials: Bases language training specifically on a child's own language patterns.

Scoring procedures: Identifies syntactic rules that a child has acquired.

Examiner qualifications and training desired: Anyone who can read the book and apply the information (it helps to have some knowledge of current linguistics).

Standard: Places a child at one of five language levels based on mean length of utterance.

Standardization sample: There are no age norms. Since this is a domain-referenced test, it should be used only to assess the child's language repertoire and not to compare a child with other children.

Major strengths: Power of this approach for domain testing of a child's behavioral repertoire is promising. One advantage is that the procedure can be administered as often as desired without invalidating the test; thus it can be used for establishing base lines and tracking progress.

Major needs: Procedures for elicitation are rather loosely defined and may result in variable results. Reliability estimates need to be established, especially where pretest and posttest applications are made for assessing behavior changes.

---

* Information supplied by test's authors.

Northwestern Syntax Screening Test*

Author: Laura L. Lee.

Publisher: Northwestern University Press, Evanston, Illinois; 1971.

Time for administration: 20 minutes.

Cost: Manual and fifty record forms, $10; fifty additional record forms, $2.50 (1977).

Purpose and nature of the test: The NSST is an individually administered test of a child's ability to comprehend and produce twenty selected grammatical structures. It is designed for children ages 3 to 7. It is a screening instrument only. Its results indicate whether a more extensive examination of a child's use of grammatical forms is warranted.

The NSST is in two parts—receptive and expressive. The receptive portion uses tasks of picture selection in response to modeled sentence-pairs that contrast by a single grammatical item. The expressive portion requires exact repetition of sentence-pairs modeled by the examiner. Separate scores for receptive and expressive portions allow comparison of a child's abilities along these two parameters.

Practical aspects: A child is scored either right or wrong in his picture selection choice (receptive) or in his repetition of the modeled sentence (expressive). Testing can be done in 20 minutes with a cooperative child, but children with language problems may take longer.

The examiner needs no special training beyond the instructions in the manual. However, interpretation of test results, decisions on the necessity for further testing, and consideration for interventional training are best done by experienced language clinicians. Information and advice on test interpretation are given in the manual.

Standardization information: Norms for ages 3-7 are given in both table and graph form. Selected percentiles (10th, 25th, 50th, 75th, and 90th) are graphed and a child's percentile for his chronological age can be estimated. Norms were based on 344 midwestern suburban children from middle and upper-middle socioeconomic homes where standard English was spoken.

It is recommended that examiners develop local norms for other geographical and socioeconomic groups since language development may be strongly influenced by these factors. Children from nonstandard dialect homes should not be evaluated by tests for language development in standard dialect.

Reliability and validity studies have not been done on the NSST. It is to be considered as a "diagnostic indicator" only, directing the examiner either to consider grammatical development within a normal range or to study it more closely with other testing materials. Recent articles by Arndt and Byrne (*JSHD, 42*:315-327, 1977) contain critical discussions of the sta-

---

* Information supplied by test's author.

tistical information on the NSST. Lee's reply in the same issue gives further advice to clinicians on interpreting NSST scores.

Major strengths: The NSST is a useful clinical tool for (1) screening large numbers of preschool or kindergarten children, (2) estimating grammatical development with a nontalkative clinical child, (3) determining whether grammatical development is a significant part of other speech problems such as articulation, fluency, or voice, and (4) estimating receptive use of grammatical structure in a child whose expressive language is unintelligible.

Major needs: The examiner must be aware that a child's performance on the twenty sentence-pairs of the NSST does not represent the full extent of his language ability. The selected items can only be considered an initial screening of a child's comprehension and production of certain early grammatical structures.

Picture Story Language Test*

Author: Helmer R. Myklebust.

Publisher: Grune & Stratton, Inc., 111 Fifth Avenue, New York, New York 10003; 1965. Published as *Development and Disorders of Written Language,* vol. 1.

Administration time: As needed; the author indicated that most children complete the story within 20 minutes.

Cost: Listed in the seventh *Mental Measurements Yearbook* as manual—$8.50; test picture—$4.75, and set of 100 four page record forms—$7.50.

General type of test: May be individually administered. Group testing is possible, but the author states that no more than eight to ten children or adults are to be tested with one picture.

Population for which designed: Both normal and handicapped from ages 7-17.

Exact domains being tested: Myklebust's major objective was the study of language, both developmentally and diagnostically. He regards written language as the most involved of the language behaviors, as it depends upon the coordination of the visual and auditory processes with the motor system for its execution. His model of this hierarchy of symbolic behaviors is included to underlie his assertion that, having been acquired last, written language is achieved only when all the preceding levels have been established. "Greater awareness of the patterns of development and the disorders of written language should provide insights into Man's total complex of behavior linguistically."

The exact domain being assessed by the PSLT is facility with the written word, thereby indicating to the examiner the developmental level of this type of verbal behavior.

Subtests and separate scores: The five scores and their subcategories are listed below.

1-3. Productivity (total words, total sentences, words per sentence)

4. Syntax (includes these error categories: word usage, word endings, and punctuation; and these error types: additions, omissions, substitutions, and word order problems).

5. Abstract-concrete dimension (expressed in five levels: meaningless-language, concrete-descriptive, concrete-imaginative, abstract-descriptive, and abstract-imaginative).

Raw scores for each category may be expressed as an age-equivalent score, as a percentile, or as a stanine.

Qualitative features of the test materials: The examiner provides age-appropriate paper and pencils, the test picture, and a test site with adequate light and space. The examiner is advised to establish rapport, maintain objectivity, and administer the following standardized directions: "Look at this

---

* Information supplied by Lynn Clapp.

picture carefully." After about a twenty-second pause, "You are to write a story about it. You may look at it as much and as often as you care to. Be sure to write the best story you can. Begin writing whenever you are ready." The examiner is advised to remain present and available but in the background. Time is given as needed. Questions during testing are answered in a neutral manner indicating that neither help nor further suggestions will be given. Encouragement is allowed in the event of an "I can't."

The objective: "To secure the best sample of written language of which the individual is capable, even if it is only a few poorly produced words or phrases."

Examiner qualifications and training: Myklebust writes that specific training in the use of this test is not essential, but that "training in the use of objectiveness as well as in the interpretation of test scores is necessary."

Normative data: This was presented in tabular form that displayed mean scores as a function of chronological age for the five areas of interest.

The PSLT was standardized on children selected from three types of public school populations: metropolitan, rural, and suburban. Within the metropolitan group, care was taken to select six schools thought to be (as judged by a group of local educators) representative as to SES and ethnicity. Total N in standardization sample = 747.

Reliability: Myklebust reported that development of a duplicate form proved to be impractical, as did immediate test-retesting. Myklebust studied interscorer reliability and found them "excellent," which translates to a range of 0.38 to 0.84 for words per sentence and a range of 0.52 to 0.92 for syntax, both at the 0.01 levels. Three of his scorers were trained, seven untrained. Reliability scores for the trained examiners were above 0.90 for total words, total sentences, and words per sentence, not at all surprising since this is a frequency task. Surprising, however, was the drop to below 0.90 in words per sentence for the untrained examiners. Reliability coefficients ranged from 0.52 to 0.91 on this task.

Interscorer reliability for the trained examiners ranged from 0.34 to 0.95, and the untrained ranged from 0.21 to 0.88; these figures apply only to the syntax score.

Validity: Myklebust acknowledges in vol. 1 that his validity data are inadequate; he claims face validity in the observation of normal children's gradually increasing proficiency with written language. Examination of his growth curves, however, indicate some nonlinearity in the upper age ranges for which no explanation was given.

Predictive validity presented some problems, in that the PSLT was unique in written projective testing. While total words, total sentences, syntax, or abstract-concrete scores were not comparable, Myklebust compared his words per sentence scores with those reported in three earlier studies and found close agreement. Other validities were not reported in vol. 1. Eight years later, in 1973, the second volume was published.

Intercorrelations among the derived scores were listed in tabular form in the second volume, but only on a portion of the urban sample; these were selected to be comparable with selected groups of handicapped children for later study, hence are not representative of the standardization sample.

Major strengths: Uniqueness. This appears to be a one-of-a-kind analysis, and —if used clinically—can offer insights into the written form of symbolization. The last half of vol. 2 is recommended reading. In this section Myklebust reports his test administration results with specific handicapped groups, including those with reading disabilities, dyslexia, mental retardation, articulatory disorders, social-emotional disturbances, and learning disabilities.

Major needs: The need for adequate reliability and validity is apparent. It may well be that these goals are unrealistic to this kind of test, which may require years of training to consistently administer and evaluate.

Porch Index of Communicative Ability in Children*

Author: Bruce E. Porch.

Publisher: Consulting Psychologists Press, 577 College Ave., Palo Alto, Calif. 94306; 1974.

Time required to administer: 45 minutes.

Cost: $52.00 (1977).

General type of test: Individual.

Population for which designed: Basic battery 3-5 years; advanced battery 6-10 years.

Exact domains being tested: General communicative ability.

Subtests and separate scores: Overall, gestural, verbal, graphic, general communication, visual, and auditory. All subtests revolve around ten common objects and therefore content is held constant and intermodality and intersubtest comparison can be made.

Qualitative features of test materials: Use of actual objects permits the testing of gestural capacity of children.

Scoring procedures: Multidimensional binary choice scoring system.

Examiner qualifications and training desired: Forty-hour training workshop plus reliability checks.

Norms: Percentiles and means.

Standardization sample: Fifty children at each age level from ages 3 to 10. The children were selected as having no history of medical, social, psychological, or educational problems; no significant speech or hearing defects, and normal intelligence. Subgroup norms are presented by age, sex, and education.

Reliability: No information given.

Validity: No information given.

Major strengths: The psychometric methods employed in this battery had been field tested in the adult form of this test for the past ten years and have been found to be extremely reliable and stable. The multidimensional binary choice scoring system quantifies each child's response in terms of five dimensions: accuracy, responsiveness, completeness, promptness, and efficiency. With the sixteen scoring categories, it is possible to describe changes in even very involved children, such as severely mentally retarded or autistic children. The use of actual stimuli and the method of using the same ten common objects through all subtests permits the tester to obtain ten homogenous samples of behavior for each subtest and it allows for more valid interpretation across subtests and between modalities.

Major needs: The PICAC as of this date (October 1, 1977) is still in its research edition. The initial data shows the test to be very reliable and stable and as soon as the normative data has been analyzed, the test will be released for general clinical use. Large N studies with the various subgroups

---

* Information supplied by test's author.

of communicative disorders in children need to be completed over the next few years to give the test full interpretive strength.

Other comments: The requirement of a forty-hour training course and periodic reliability checks is an inconvenience for the clinician but is necessary if the test is to be used appropriately.

Preschool Language Scale*

Authors: Irla Lee Zimmerman, Violette Steiner, and Roberta Evatt Pond.

Publisher: C. E. Merrill Company, 1300 Alum Creek Drive, Columbus, Ohio 43216; 1969.

Administration time: 15-25 minutes.

Cost: Complete package (manual, picture book, record booklets) $7.95; record booklets (10) $4.95 (1977).

Type: Individually administered language scale.

Population: Children suspected of language deficits or deficiencies in their native or second language, and assumed to be functioning linguistically below 7 years of age. Specific populations include culturally deprived and/or language deficient children such as those enrolled in Head Start, bilingual, and other compensatory programs, as well as hospitalized and institutionalized children who are assumed to have linguistic impairment or language retardation.

Exact domains: The level of present language functioning in the areas of receptive and expressive language skills. The former is measured nonverbally, while the latter requires verbal responses.

Subtests and separate scores: The scale is composed of two distinct sections permitting separate assessment of auditory comprehension (receptive) and verbal ability, including articulation (expressive), each measured by forty items covering the language ages 2 through 7. An overall language age score is obtained by averaging the auditory-comprehension and verbal-ability age scores. The three language age scores can be converted to language quotients for comparison purposes.

Practical aspects: Qualitative features of test materials: A colorful thirty-two-page picture book appealing to children and a few simple objects, such as colored blocks, easily assessible to individuals in a school or similar environment. A record booklet contains all test questions and allows the examiner sufficient room to record full responses, and to score and identify specific strengths and weaknesses.

Scoring procedures: Items are scored plus or minus according to age-established criteria. Examples are provided in the manual. The sum of items passed provide a language age score.

Examiner qualifications: Speech therapists, psychologists, and qualified school personnel including teachers who are trained and supervised by psychologists and/or speech therapists.

Standardization information: Item placement, established by various authorities through studies of language development, was verified by item analysis of some 300 Head Start, mentally retarded, language handicapped, and normal preschool and kindergarten children. Because of the experimental nature of the scale, norms are not given in the test manual. How-

---

* Information supplied by test's authors.

ever the manual and scale are being revised to incorporate current standardization studies. The need to incorporate changes in child development has been established by the recent restandardization of the Stanford Binet and Wechsler Intelligence Scale for Children.

Reliability: Reliability data have been collected using the split-half method with correction for length of the test by the Spearman-Brown formula. Reliability coefficients obtained for two consecutive years of Head Start classes ranged from 0.75 to 0.92, median 0.88.

Validity: Concurrent validity studies are available, covering comparisons of the Preschool Language Scale with the Illinois Test of Psycholinguistics, the Peabody Picture Vocabulary Test, the Utah Test of Language Development, and the Stanford Binet, among others. Predictive studies using the Lee Clark Reading Readiness Test indicated that the Preschool Language Scale predicted reading success for two thirds of the children studied.

Major Strengths:

1. Simple, rapid administration and scoring.
2. Presents both receptive and expressive language competencies in readily understood terms.
3. Allows for the identification of specific language strengths, lags, or deficiencies. On this basis the professional educator, clinician, or therapist can plan effective individual and group language learning programs.
4. Pretesting and posttesting of children permit evaluation of the effectiveness of language training programs, while attention can also be directed to areas calling for further intervention.
5. Provides a method for comparing children's ability to verbalize and articulate with their level of language comprehension, in order to assess the need of and readiness for speech therapy.
6. In its various forms, the Preschool Language Scale permits testing, evaluation, and comparison of English, as well as other language (to date, Spanish, French, and Inupiate) status of preschool or language disabled children and facilitates understanding of their language needs. This minimizes either overestimating or underestimating actual language skills, and clarifies the status of children in bilingual programs by identifying the language best suited for beginning formal instruction.

Major needs: Revision of the manual and scale (now underway) to include current normative data and reliability and validity studies.

Other comments: Printed reviews.

Jackson, C. H. Review of the Preschool Language Scale. *Journal and Newsletter Association of Educational Psychologists,* 2:5, 1970.

Proger, B. B. Review of the Preschool Language Scale. *Journal of Special Education,* 5:85-85, 1971.

Reynell Developmental Language Scales*

Author: Joan K. Reynell.

Publisher and date: NFER Publishing Co., Ltd., Darville House, 2 Oxford Road East, Windsor S14 1DF, England; 1977.

Brief description: This test is given individually and takes about one-half hour to administer. Cost breakdowns for the test are as follows (1977): complete set—$87.50; manual—$10.50; thirty-five record forms—$17.50; kit of toys and pictures come only with the complete set.

The test was designed to be used with children between the ages of 1 and 6 years. It consists of three subtests, each generating independent scores (total test scores were not standardized): (1) Verbal Comprehension A; (2) Verbal Comprehension B; and (3) Expressive Language. Verbal Comprehension subtest B was designed especially for use with children with limited response repertoires. The use of the test is restricted to clinical or educational psychologists, speech therapists, and those who have completed a special course of training in use of the test.

Standardization information: Age-equivalent values, means, standard deviations, and standard scores are available for each subtest at each of twelve different age levels. Samples for standardization were comprised of 1,318 children (662 boys and 656 girls) aged 1 to 7 years from the southern, middle, and northern parts of England. 903 children were tested on the first stage of revision, and 415 children were tested on the final stage of revision; these data were then combined for inclusion in the normative tables.

Reliability: Split-half correlation coefficients were calculated for each of the twelve age levels; range of reliability coefficients for ages 1.5 through 5.5 years was 0.81 to 0.96 (range for the total group was 0.46 to 0.96).

Validity: No validity studies have been reported.

Major strengths: This test can be efficiently administered, it gives developmental information, and makes special provisions for children with restricted response repertoires.

Major needs: Not all of the normative-sample children were tested on all of the subtests; it would be helpful if a single test score could be provided to give an overall index of language development.

---

* Information supplied by test's publisher.

Structured Photographic Language Test*

Authors: Ellen O'Hara Werner and Janet Dawson Krescheck.

Publisher, date of publication: Janelle Publications, P.O. Box 12, Sandwich, Illinois 60548; June 1977.

Time required to administer: 15 to 25 minutes.

Cost: $30.00—includes test manual, fifty-one colored photographs, one response form, one languagegram, one language profile sheet. $5.00—twenty-five response forms. $5.00—twenty-five languagegrams and twenty-five language profile sheets.

General type of test: The purpose of the Structured Photographic Language Test is to assess the child's formulation of critical morphophonemic and syntactic structures. The child is required to generate a specific structure in response to controlled auditory and visual stimuli which provides the context for the response. The test is administered on an individual basis.

Population for which designed: Male and female, black and white, children from 4.0 to 8.11 years of age.

Exact domains being tested: The following lists the specific syntactic structures and forms that are elicited and thus scored. (There are fifty-one items.)

1. Prepositional phrases.
2. Singular noun.
3. Plural nouns /z/, /s/, /ez/.
4. Third person singular present tense or present progressive tense, regular and irregular verbs.
5. Future or present progressive plus infinitive ("to" + verb), regular and irregular verbs.
6. Past tense, regular and irregular verbs.
7. Third person plural present tense or present progressive tense, regular and irregular verbs.
8. Past tense, regular, copulas.
9. Infinitive complements.
10. Imperatives.
11. Negative imperative.
12. Conjunction *and* joining two sentences.
13. Conjunction *because* joining two sentences or solely initiating second sentence in response to *Why?*
14. Conjunction *and*.
15. Possessive nouns.
16. Possessive pronouns yours, your, mine, my, hers, her.
17. Participles.
18. Infinitive used with a subject differing from the main subject.
19. Negatives.
20. Passive with *was* or *got*.

---

* Information supplied by test's authors.

21. Reflexive pronouns, *himself, myself.*
22. *Yes/no* interrogatives.
23. *Wh* questions, Case I.
24. *Wh* questions, Case II.
25. *Wh* questions, Case III.
26. Negative *Wh* question.

Qualitative features of test materials: The SPLT requires no special training in linguistics for either administration or scoring.

Full color photographs of children, adults, and animals in everyday situations paired with brief storylike statements are the stimulus materials used to elicit each structure. This procedure permits the child to generate structures that might be omitted in a more unstructured sample while avoiding duplication of structures. The scoring procedure allows the examiner to distinguish those children who perform substantially below others of their age.

The controlled corpus of utterances permits comparison of child's productions with others of his geographical and socioeconomic environment. The SPLT also provides a system of alternative response structures for assessment of children who use black English. An explanation of the rules of black English is included.

Scoring procedures: The test items are scored as correct or incorrect. The total number of correct responses is tabulated and a percent correct score is found. A graph that displays the scores and standard deviation shows sufficient problems in producing grammatical structures to warrant enrollment in therapy or further evaluation. For a child whose score falls below the second standard deviation on the test, a suggested, but optional, method of analyzing his productions is presented using a languagegram and language profile sheet.

The languagegram shows the age at which 90 percent of the children tested correctly produced each item. The language profile sheet summarizes the child's performance.

Norms: Mean percent correct and standard deviations are given for ten age groups.

Standardization sample: The test was standardized on 360 children between the ages of 4.0 and 8.11 years. These children came from middle socioeconomic classes where standard American English was the sole language spoken. All children were selected from preschools and public schools in the Chicago suburbs and other communities in northern Illinois. These children were of normal intelligence with no evident speech or hearing problems as determined by the clinical judgment of a qualified clinician.

Reliability: Test-retest reliability: Twenty children (four each at four, five, six, seven, and eight year age levels) were selected at random, tested, and retested within ten days from the first administration of the test. The

Pearson product-moment correlation coefficient obtained was 0.95, denoting highly consistent results.

Validity: Analysis of data of twenty-five children who were diagnosed as language delayed by the SPLT also were diagnosed as significantly language delayed by the DSS method. Further, the data obtained thus far follow for the most part of the patterns of language development found in the literature. Many of the age norms for the structures on the languagegram are in keeping with developmental age levels found in the literature on normal language acquisition. Percents of total correct responses also increased with age.

Major strengths: The test permits a child's expressive formulation of critical syntactic structures, while controlling the elicitation techniques, instructions, and stimulus material. The test has been designed to quickly allow the examiner to distinguish those children who perform substantially below others of their age in the production of grammatical structures. The test provides a system of alternative response structures for assessment of black children. The test provides a means of making a detailed analysis of all the utterances a child generates in response to the stimuli.

Major needs: Additional validity data showing concurrent relationship of test scores with spontaneous performance in unstructured situations would be helpful.

System Fore: Developmental Language Program*

Author: Division of Special Education, Los Angeles Unified School District.

Publisher, date of publication: Division of Special Education, Los Angeles Unified School District; 1972.

Time required to administer: 30-45 minutes (depending on level of pupil).

Cost: $16.00; order from Speech and Language Unit, 6651 Balboa Blvd., Van Nuys, California 91406.

General type of test: May be administered individually or in small groups.

Population for which designed: Birth to 10 years (Level 0 through Level 13).

Exact domains being tested: Phonology, morphology, syntax, and semantics.

Subtests and separate scores: Spanish adaptations: A Spanish translation of levels 3 through 10 is used to assess language levels of monolingual Spanish-speaking children ages 3-7 years.

Qualitative features of test materials: Establishes a language profile to show strengths and weaknesses in the four linguistic strands: phonology, morphology, syntax, and semantics.

Scoring procedures: Individual and group scoring procedures are included.

Examiner qualifications and training desired: Speech and language specialist, classroom teacher.

Norms: This is a nonstandardized inventory arranged sequentially according to child development levels. This domain-referenced test may be used in assessing speech and language skills by the speech and language specialist, the classroom teacher, or both in a team approach. It is designed as a classroom management system for planning an individualized instructional program for pupils.

Validity: An item analysis tested the validity of objectives and inventory items at selected developmental levels.

The inventories were administered by speech and language specialists to pupils whose birthdates correlated with developmental age levels of the language sequences to test suitability and clarity of test items and directions.

Size and nature of samples employed: 58 boys and 58 girls (126 pupils), kindergarten-third, from a range of socioeconomic areas were tested.

Major strengths: The Developmental Language Program has four components:

1. The developmental language sequences are arranged according to child developmental levels, beginning at birth (level 0) and continuing to 10 years (level 18).

2. This language program contains a criterion-referenced inventory with which to assess mastery levels of pupils in each of four linguistic areas: phonology, morphology, syntax, and semantics.

---

* Information supplied by test's publisher.

3. A record keeping system has been designed to record individual student responses or group response for classroom use.
4. The instructional materials information list suggests appropriate material and equipment correlated with the language sequences by strand, level, and item. These four components comprise the classroom management system.

Major needs: Time to administer the inventories may pose a problem.

Other comments: System FORE: Developmental Language Program assists the teacher to develop specific instructional objectives for each pupil, plan units of instruction at appropriate levels for each pupil, record pupil performance, group pupils for instruction, write an educational plan (IEP/IIP) for each pupil.

Test of Auditory Comprehension of Language

Author: Elizabeth Carrow-Woodfolk.

Publisher, date of publication: Learning Concepts, 2501 North Lamar, Austin, Texas 78705; 1973.

Time required to administer: 20-30 minutes.

Cost: $39.95 (1978).

General type of test: Individual.

Population for which designed: 3.0 to 6.11 years.

Exact domains being tested: Auditory comprehension of vocabulary and linguistic structures.

Subtests and separate scores: Vocabulary, morphology, and syntax.

Qualitative features of test materials: Manual of instructions, 101 reusable picture stimuli, 3-ring vinyl binder, 25 scoring forms.

Scoring procedures: Child responds to examiner's oral stimuli in English or Spanish by pointing to one of three line drawings.

Examiner qualifications and training desired: BA in education, psychology, or sociology and considerable testing experience.

Norms: Percentile ranks and age-score equivalents.

Standardization sample: 200 middle-class black, Anglo-American, and Mexican-American children between the ages of 3 and 6 years.

Reliability. Test-retest correlation coefficients of 0.93 and 0.94 for English and Spanish versions respectively.

Validity: Construct and criterion-related validity are presented. Test scores discriminate between normal and linguistically handicapped and increase significantly with age of child.

Major strengths: Convenient, easily managed, and quick to administer.

Major needs: Normative data need to be made available for the Spanish version.

Utah Test of Language Development

Authors: M. J. Mecham, J. L. Jex, and J. D. Jones.

Publisher: Communication Research Associates, Inc., P.O. Box 11013, Salt Lake City, Utah 84147; 1978 revised edition.

Brief description: This test is administered individually and takes about 20 to 30 minutes. Kit costs $35.00 (includes manual, picture plates, objects, twenty-five score sheets, and a custom designed carrying case). It was designed to be used with children between the ages of 1.5 years and 14 years. It assesses functional use of language for communication; such functional use involves knowledge of semantic and syntactic structures but these aspects are not evaluated as entities separated from functional use. The test can therefore be used only as a diagnostic screening test.

Testing begins with each child at a level just a little under his C.A.; items are tested downward until eight consecutive pluses are obtained, and then upward above the starting point until eight consecutive minuses are obtained—at which point the test is discontinued. Items are scored as correct (plus) or incorrect (minus). The total score is the total number of items passed; it indicates the chronological age standard score equivalents of the child's language development.

The test must be administered by professional clinicians or teachers who have had previous training in standardized testing. Thorough familiarity with the test is required (thorough familiarity with test instructions, scoring procedures, etc.) and prior practice in administering the test is essential.

Standardization information: Mean scores and standard deviations for each of thirteen different age levels are provided, as are standard and percentile scores. Level of language development is estimated from chronological age level equivalent values for various raw scores. The normative group was comprised of 666 children fairly equally distributed over various age levels (about one-half boys and one-half girls at each level. 273 of the norm group were represented by an equal number of subjects from each of three socioeconomic levels, i.e. upper-lower, lower-middle, and middle. The remaining 393 were selected unsystematically from twenty-three different states in the United States (95 percent were white and 5 percent were black).

Additionally, a group of 989 kindergarten children, selected randomly from the Salt Lake City schools, were tested and their scores were converted into percentiles. This group was comprised of 83.8 percent Caucasians, 0.7 percent American Indians, 11.9 percent Chicanos, 1.3 percent Orientals, and 2.2 percent blacks.

Reliability: The UTLD and the Verbal Language Development Scale (an indirect test version of the UTLD) were administered to 117 normal children and a correlation coefficient was computed on resulting scores; the

Pearson Product Moment correlation coefficient was 0.967. These two alternate forms were also administered to forty institutionalized mentally retarded subjects; the resulting correlation coefficient was 0.810.

Internal consistency of the UTLD was estimated by use of the Kuder-Richardson formula 21 on the original 272 normative subjects. The resulting correlation coefficient was 0.870.

Validity: Validity of the UTLD was checked by the method of calibration. First, since all items of the scale had been selected previously from standardized sources, it was felt that the items had good "face" validity. One way of checking the agreement between the UTLD normative data and the original item sources was to correlate the chronological age equivalents of the UTLD norms and the norms from the original sources. Product-moment correlation of ages of items in the UTLD sample with their age levels in the original tests was 0.983.

Item validity was checked by correlating each item on the test with total test scores. All items except item one were well over 0.40 in discrimination power. This suggests acceptable validity in terms of item discrimination power.

Some research has been undertaken relative to concurrent validity. One study revealed a correlation coefficient between the UTLD and the Illinois Test of Psycholinguistic Abilities on twenty-five mentally retarded subjects to be 0.912: in another study, the UTLD and ITPA were administered to eleven mentally retarded children and the resulting rank correlation coefficient was 0.870.

Major strengths. The UTLD is easy to administer; it is a sensitive measure of level of language development and an indicator of where to begin in training. Preliminary data suggest that the total score does not reflect significant cultural bias. Small groups of questions from the test can be administered in 5 minutes or less for quick screening with a fairly high degree of reliability and validity.

Major need: Additional research on content and concurrent validity would be of value.

Vane Evaluation of Language Scale
(The Vane-L): An Achievement Measure
for Young Children 2.5 to 6 years*

Author: Julia R. Vane.

Publisher: Published as monograph no. 49, *Archives of the Behavioral Sciences,* September 1975.

Available from: Clinical Psychology Publishing Co., Inc., 4 Conant Square, Brandon, Vermont 05733.

Administration time: 10-15 minutes.

Cost: Vane-L manual—$5.00; test kit—$8.00; package of fifty test blanks—$3.50; complete package—$15.00.

General type of test: Individually administered screening scale that assesses both receptive and expressive language.

Population for which designed: Children from 2.5 to 6 years.

Exact domains being tested: Receptive and expressive language. Additionally, handedness and attention (memory) may be measured.

Subtests and separate scores: Percentile equivalents are given for receptive scores, expressive scores, and memory scores for eight age groups within the age range of 2-6 to 6-5 years.

The receptive language domain includes knowledge of body parts, action words, and singular-plural distinctions. A point is given each correct response to direct commands using the child's own body parts, the bottles and beans, the blocks and cars, to the test item box container itself, and to each of the thirty-eight concepts tested.

The expressive language domain includes responses to requests for self-identifying information, a sentence repetition task that ranges from two-word sentences, and an estimate of vocabulary through asking "What is a ———? or What does ——— mean?" A point is given for each entirely correct response in the information and sentence-repetition tasks. Samples of scoring each of the ten vocabulary words are given, and each is scored 2, 1, or 0 points.

The memory domain is two-fold: The earlier sentence repetition is included as an attempt to measure auditory verbal memory, and the child is able to score twice on this task. The task is seen as involving skill in both repetitive accuracy and memory.

The second memory task is successful imitation of the examiner's concealed block tapping pattern. This is scored as an auditory motor memory task; however, if the child is unable to accurately repeat the tapping pattern using auditory cues alone, the tasks may be repeated while the child is allowed to watch. Comparisons are made of his auditory, visual, and auditory + visual responses on the increasingly complex tasks, but he is scored only on his first trial.

---

* Information supplied by Lynn Clapp.

Additional observations regarding hand preference in a specified number of trials may be recorded.

Qualitative features of test materials: Packed in a compact, sturdy 11″ × 2.5″ × 3″ corrugated cardboard box. Unbreakable materials include seven clear-stained, smooth-wooden blocks in four sizes; two small plastic cars with no removable parts, red and blue and pliable; and five hard-surfaced, clear plastic cylinders securely glued to a sanded, red-painted wooden base. Four of the cylinders contain dried beans; the fifth is unsealed and empty. Test blanks contain administration directions, are clearly printed and well organized, and arranged with a face sheet containing identifying information, subscores, and percentile scores.

Scoring procedures: One point for each item throughout. Vocabulary section scored 2, 1, 0 points as directed.

Examiner qualifications: Employment in preschools or kindergartens. Practice on another adult or child above seven years of age is recommended. "It is not recommended that the scale be given to a child, for whom it is to be used as a diagnostic tool, without reading the manual completely."

Standardization information: The 740 children in the standardization group were drawn from many areas in three states—New York, New Jersey, and Vermont. They were tested by psychologists trained in testing children, and tested under conditions that "approximate the conditions under which most children are tested." The author intended to have her standardization sample conform to the 1970 United States census data with respect to age, sex, race (white/nonwhite), occupation of parent, and urban/rural residence. She reports that her results included successful distribution according to parental occupation, but a bias was reported in the urban direction (only 12 percent of the sample was drawn from the rural areas as compared with 22 percent in the country as a whole and no children of farmers or farm laborers were included). Few children from very large inner cities were tested, but poverty areas from cities with populations of about 60,000 were "adequately sampled." Geographical areas included were limited to three northeastern states. The author cautions the user that her N of children from 2.5 to 3 years is small and that norms for this group should be considered tentative. She decided to reject the option of including the noncooperative 2-year-olds with zero scores, thereby increasing sample size, but lowering the norms for this age cluster.

Reliability: Data were not included in the manual.

Validity: Content validity. Selection of items for the Vane-L was based upon the administration of different forms to over 2,000 children ranging in age from 2-6 years over a four-year period. The scale underwent many changes as a result of this field testing to control for the operation of chance, to control for the children's predispositional sets, and to aid in ease of administration. Particular attention was paid to the elimination of class bias in the selection of vocabulary items, but item analysis revealed that middle-class children knew more of these words than lower-class children of the same age with the exception of the word *hungry*. Lower-class children defined this word accurately more often than middle-class children of the same age. The author does not cite publication of this data in her bibliography, however.

Intercorrelations of the various subtests at each age level with one another and the total expressive and receptive sections were presented in tabular form. They ranged from $+0.48$ to $+0.71$ at all age levels for expressive and receptive, but the correlations were not so high as to suggest that the same areas of language were being assessed. The author acknowledges that the high correlation (ranging between 0.93 and 0.98) of the concept subtest to the total receptive section reflects the heavy weighting of the receptive section with the concept items—as does, to a lesser degree, the weighting of the expressive section with the vocabulary subtest. Tapping, which is a "measure of nonverbal memory," showed no consistent relation to any of the other subtests with the exception of sentences, another measure of memory. The correlation between taps and sentences was in the low positive range of 0.23 to 0.48. This combined with the fact that sentences correlate in a high positive fashion to the total expressive section and within the same range to the total receptive section suggests that memory assessed by the sentences is strongly dependent upon language facility, but that memory assessed by taps is independent of language facility.

Criterion-related validity. The author reports low correlations between the Vane Kindergarten Test, which measures intellectual ability, and the Vane-L scores, and asserts that these low correlations suggest that the tests are measuring something different.

Predictive validity. The Vane-L was administered as a pretest and again as a posttest at the end of a school year to 166 preschoolers. Tabular data reveal that these 166 children scored below the Vane-L norms on the pretest. Gains were recorded as means, Vane-L norms, deviations from norms, raw score gains, and norm gains for children in morning and afternoon classes with five teachers. Vane suggests one possible use of this scale would be for the development of local norms, which may be more useful to schools than standardized norms.

Major strengths: Ease of administration, high interest in materials and interaction with administrator, quick screen for conceptual strengths, singular-plural markers, body parts, action words, general information, sentence repetition, and vocabulary are felt to be strengths of this test. It is possible to estimate interactional skills, dexterity, and attending behaviors in addition to the language skills tapped.

Major needs: Reliability studies would be helpful since the confidence one places in validity reports is contingent upon a satisfactory degree of reliability.

Verbal Language Development Scale

Author: Merlin J. Mecham.

Publisher: American Guidance Service, Publishers Bldg., Circle Pines, Minnesota 55014; 1971 revised edition.

Brief description: Testing time is approximately 15 minutes. Cost of the test is ninety cents for the manual and $2.35 for twenty-five score sheets (1977). The test is administered individually and is designed to be used with children between the ages of 0 and 16 years.

It assesses functional use of language for communication. It yields a single score but gives indications of possible problems in listening, speaking, reading, and writing as specific domains.

It is an informant-interview type test; the score is based on descriptions given by a knowledgeable reporter. Three types of scoring are used—plus (established behaviors), plus-minus (partially established), and minus (unestablished behaviors). The test should be administered only by professional clinicians and teachers who have had training in standardized testing. Complete familiarity with item definitions and scoring procedures is required.

Standardization information: Mean scores and their chronological age equivalent levels are presented in tabular form; a total score is interpreted in terms of chronological age equivalent as established by the norm-group data. The norm group was comprised of 273 normal white children (119 boys and 118 girls) selected in approximately equal numbers from fourteen different age levels; the normative subjects were selected to represent the three predominant SES levels, i.e. upper-lower, lower-middle, and middle.

Reliability: Correlation of this scale with the UTLD (equivalent form) on 117 normal children was 0.970; correlations of the two tests on 40 educable mentally retarded children was 0.720, and with 45 trainable mentally retarded children was 0.810. Test-retest correlation coefficient with 28 mentally retarded subjects was 0.960.

Validity: Concurrent validity was suggested by a correlation coefficient of 0.930 between this scale and the Stanford Binet, Form L, on 92 mentally retarded subjects: correlation coefficient of this scale with the Peabody Picture Vocabulary Test was 0.790 on 22 mentally retarded subjects. Correlation of scores on this scale and the ratings of extent of language delay by eleven competent clinicians on 92 mentally retarded subjects 0.940.

Construct validity was supported by a study in which two groups of deaf students, one with high and one with low intelligence scores on the WISC were matched as to degree of hearing loss and C.A. Scores of the high and low intelligence groups did not differ significantly on this scale, suggesting that this scale does not measure intelligence per se.

Major strengths: This test is a quick, reliable screening tool that can be used conveniently with hard to test subjects, such as aphasic, hyperactive, or autistic children. It gives an estimate of level of language development and of the point at which training should begin.

Major needs: Expanded norms need to be acquired in order that standard scores or percentiles can be made available.

Vocabulary Comprehension Scale
Pronouns and Words of Position, Size, Quality, and Quantity*

Author: Tina E. Bangs.

Publisher: Learning Concepts, 2501 N. Lamar, Austin Texas 78705.

Date: November 1972.

Cost: Kit = $39.00, fifty response forms = $8.00 (1977).

Population for which designed: 2.0 to 6.0 years.

Domains being tested: Assesses comprehensive vocabulary appropriate for entrance into kindergarten or first grade; specifically, pronouns and words of position, size, quality, and quantity.

Practical aspects:

   (1) Objects as test materials rather than pictures.

   (2) Different scenes used, presorted according to domain tested.

   (3) Scoring procedures:

      a. Examiner statement for each vocabulary item tested is given on score sheet. Example: "Take the car *out* of the garage."

      b. Score is pass (+) or fail (−); blank if not administered.

      c. Child must name or point to all objects used in scale.

      d. Examiner makes judgment regarding test termination.

      e. No gestures are used by examiner; no indication of failure is to be given; praise given as needed.

      f. Directions may be repeated if child requests or if examiner feels it is necessary.

      g. Credit is given for two out of three correct responses on all test items. (Note: scoring instructions do not advise elsewhere that items may be repeated if child fails—this must be assumed from the credit statement.)

      h. When testing opposites, objects are to be randomly presented to alternating hands.

Testing time: Not given.

Examiner qualifications and training desired: Not stated.

Norms:

   a. Population defined and described: 80 children from low-middle to high-middle income homes, of mixed ethnic backgrounds, enrolled in preschool programs in Houston, Texas, preselected by classroom teacher, and no obvious language deficits.

   b. Sampling method: Children chosen on basis of PPVT score (at, above, or no more than six months below age level were accepted for study); no discussion of possible bias given in manual.

   c. Size of sample: Ten children in each six-month age level between 2.0 and 6.0 years. Total = 80 children. (Information regarding ethnic mix,

---

* Information supplied by Jane M. Carpenter.

sex, educational status given above, no further information given in manual.)

d. Conditions: Examiners included author and two persons trained by her.

Data analysis:

a. Cutoff points between 80-100 percent correct responses.

b. Each level selected was point at which 80 percent of subjects comprehended the words.

c. This criteria had to be met at successive age levels.

Ages:	2.0	2.6	3.0	3.6
	2.6	3.0	3.6	4.0
"soft":	3/10	8/10	8/10	9/10

d. Exceptions: Words *less, their,* and *different* met criteria at lower age level, then slipped below 8/10 requirement at later age levels. Lower score was used and teachers cautioned that these words may not be stable.

Reliability: No information given.

Validity: No information given.

Comments: Author states:

a. "Child's semantic knowledge is basic to his success in kindergarten and first grade." No rationale given for selection of these particular words, especially pronouns.

b. Author suggests that classroom teacher organize special lesson plans designed to teach words and concepts unfamiliar to child, i.e. words failed on the test.

c. Author suggested lesson plans are included in manual for speech therapist, classroom teacher, and parents.

d. Appendix A gives interpretative age level norms for each word tested.

e. Appendix B lists materials included in test.

f. Appendix C gives percentage of students meeting criterion for each word at six-month age intervals.

Major strengths: This test taps the child's knowledge of selected cognitively oriented labels that are assessed in the context of a play situation. It is relatively easy to administer and is likely to stimulate a high level of interest in young children.

Major needs: Expanded norms and studies of reliability and validity would enable clinicians to know something about the usefulness of this test for formal testing.

References

Buros, O. K.: *The seventh mental measurements yearbook.* Highland Park, N. J.: Gryphon Press, 1972.

Clark, P. M.: *System FORE: Developmental language program.* Van Nuys, California: Los Angeles Unified School District, 1972.

Cronbach, L. J.: *Essentials of psychological testing (3rd ed.).* New York: Har-Row, 1970.

Darley, F. L., Siegel, G. M., Fay, W. M., Newman, P. W., and Rees, M. (Eds.): *Evaluation of assessment techniques in speech pathology.* New York: Addison-Wesley (in press).

Donlon, T. F.: Referencing test scores: introductory concepts. In Hively, W., and Reynolds, M. C. (Eds.), *Domain-referenced testing in special education.* Reston, Va.: The Council for Exceptional Children, 1975.

Gronlund, N. E.: *Preparing criterion-referenced tests for classroom instruction.* New York: Macmillan, 1973.

Gronlund, N. E.: *Construction of achievement tests.* Englewood Cliffs, New Jersey: P-H, 1977.

Guilford, J.: *The nature of human intelligence.* New York: McGraw, 1967.

Junker, K. S.: *Selective attention in infants and consecutive communicative behavior.* Stockholm: Almqvist and Wiksell, 1972.

Hersen, M. and Barlow, D. H.: *Single case experimental designs: Strategies for studying behavior change.* New York: Pergamon Press, 1976.

Porch, B. E.: *Porch index of communicative ability in children.* Palo Alto, California: Consulting Psychologists, 1974.

Siegel, S.: *Nonparametric statistics for the behavioral sciences.* New York: McGraw, 1956.

Sternberg, S.: Memory-scanning: Mental processes revealed by reaction-time experiments. *Am Sci, 57:*421-457, 1969.

Stillman, R. D.: *Assessment of deaf-blind children: The Collier-Azusa scale.* Reston, Virginia: The Council for Exceptional Children, 1974.

Uzgiris, I. C. and IIunt, J. McV.: *Assessment in infancy.* Urbana, Illinois: U of Ill Pr, 1975.

Warren, R. L., Hubbard, D. I., and Knox, A. W.: Short-term memory scan in normal individuals and individuals with aphasia. *J Speech Hear Res, 20:* 497-509, 1977.

Chapter 4

INFORMAL ASSESSMENT OF LANGUAGE DISORDERS

T HROUGH THE USE of valid and reliable tests where certain language skills of a child may be compared with normative data, the speech clinician can determine if a child has a significant language problem. However, the complete description of a child's language behavior will involve additional informal measures. Informal measures include evaluations that are based on knowledge and experience but are not standardized. Although not standardized, when carefully planned and executed these informal procedures augment formal language testing in a complete language assessment.

Informal measures should be undertaken with organized planning to suit the individual child. These informal descriptions of a child's language and associated behaviors should have the direct purpose of providing data that will enable the clinician to develop a treatment plan for each child. In other words, formal language testing provides the necessary comparisons to normative data but seldom provides a guide to treatment. The informal procedures in this chapter are suggested as indices of specific language problems in individuals and as guides to individual therapeutic planning.

A combination of clinical observations and elicitation and analysis of language and associated behaviors is necessary. However, some procedures are only necessary for certain children's evaluation while others are important for the assessment of each child with a language problem.

Indvidual Communicative Ability and Methods

The clinician needs to have some idea how each child communicates. In this initial informal assessment, the clinician needs to focus attention on the general communication skills of the child. Communication involves a speaker and a listener; thus the concern is a continuum of speaker-listener relationships involving the following:

1. Relationships to humans (from no recognition of another person all the way to warm relationships with other people appropriate for the age of the child).
2. Efforts in communication as a speaker (from no attempt to gesture all the way to verbalization appropriate to age level or more advanced).
3. Efforts in communication as a listener (from no attempt, to merely responding to sounds, all the way to understanding appropriate to age level or more advanced).
4. Enjoyment of communication (from no apparent desire to talk or listen all the way to enjoying talking or listening to anyone or any group).

The child's general abilities in communication and the methods he uses may be gleaned both from interviews with informants and direct observations.

An initial interview with the child's parent and/or teacher is an informative beginning point. The clinician may well begin with a sequence of questions such as the following: "How does Johnny let you know when he wants something?" "Describe what he does to get what he wants." "Suppose that Johnny wanted a cookie, tell me what he would typically do or say to you to let you know what he wanted." "Suppose Johnny doesn't want to go to bed, how would he let you know?" "How does Johnny respond to your requests?" "Tell me some typical directions, commands, or questions that he meaningfully obeys or answers." Questions along this line should tell the clinician something about the child's method of communicating with adults. Other questions should indicate the child's method of communicating with peers: "Does Sally play with other children?" "How does Sally tell her friends what she wants?" If the child is in preschool years, the clinician might ask, "Does Sally talk when she is playing alone?" When a parent or teacher indicates that the child certainly communicates by talking but they are concerned about the way a child talks, then other questions become necessary. The following might be such questions: "Tell me what you are concerned about in the way Susie talks. Tell me some things she says."

Answers provided by parents or teachers should give the clinician a general idea of the child's abilities and method of communication as seen by adults in the child's environment. However, a clinician needing to plan language treatment should also use this interview to find out what the child needs or wants to talk about in his daily life. For the preschool child, the clinician needs to know what are the child's favorite toys and books, what are the names of his family members and friends, and what foods and beverages the child likes and wants to ask for. In addition, it might be wise to find out about any toys or foods the child is not allowed to have. For instance, in some homes guns (toys or real) are not present. Likewise candy or coffee may not be available. If a clinician can determine these things it becomes apparent they will not be immediate communication needs of the child and may have no current meaning. For older children, it is valuable to find out current interests and hobbies as well as things the child does with family or friends.

Gleaning maximum information necessary for a language assessment from parents while managing to keep the parents at ease, relaxed, and confident should be the goal of the clinician in the initial interview. Bangs (1968, pp. 71-83) and Emerick and Hatten (1974, pp. 23-43) present helpful discussion on techniques of parent interviewing.

The clinician should not depend solely on others' reports of the child's ability or methods of communication. Many direct observations by the clinician throughout the entire evaluation of the child will be necessary. The clinician will want to notice how or if the child relates to his parents, the clinicians, strangers, and, if possible, peers or siblings in the halls, the office, or the waiting room. Does the child look at people; does he indicate an interest in the people and activities in the environment? Does he communicate with people and what method does he use? If he is nonverbal, is he using gestures or jargon? If he is talking, to whom is he talking and what is he saying? Opportunities will be present to observe if the child responds to greetings, directions, and questions meaningfully and in what manner.

Berry (1969, p. 201) provides a guide for noting the young or low language level child's attitude toward communication. She suggests observing such things as whether the child makes no attempt to communicate, pantomines much of the time, has excessive verbal output, is ready to initiate speech as a means of communication, and attends readily to the speech of others. A guide for assessing the communicative ability of children from upper elementary levels is provided in Lundsteen (1976, pp. 435-437). She includes the interaction process of speaker and listener and the evolution from egocentric to nonegocentric communication. For instance, she suggests that the egocentric speaker codes events so that they are meaningful for the speaker and the speaker sends the listener the events as the speaker saw them. On the other hand the nonegocentric speaker tries to alter the message to be what the listener might consider relevant.

These measures should give the clinician an idea of whether the individual child is communicating, his method of communicating, and his general ability to receive or deliver a message. In addition, some estimate may be made of the child's pleasure in the art of communication.

Developmental Observation

Another type of informal assessment should begin with the initial interview and continue throughout the evaluation process. The alert clinician uses every moment to note what the child is doing developmentally. The purpose of developmental observations should be directed toward what the clinician needs to know in order to plan treatment for the child.

The clinician should know what is to be expected developmentally of children of various age levels. Familiarity with developmental observations will demonstrate the general level of the child, which will help provide a guide for treatment, and familiarity with expected developmental stages will enable a clinician to organize observations.

For instance, observing the general coordination of the child as he takes off his coat or as he walks down the hall, or whether he climbs stairs with alternating feet will tell a clinician something about the general motor development of the child. Also observations about whether handedness is established, how the child holds a crayon or pencil, whether the child can draw or write will all provide more evidence. Using guides, the clinician can have a written or mental list of observations appropriate to the various age levels. Tables of important developmental milestones may be found in Knobloch and Pasamanick (1974). The clinician may also find the charts in Eisenson (1972) and Lenneberg (1967) that compare motor development and language development to be quite useful.

All of these observations may provide indirect input for the assessment of the child. However, often less obvious to the clinician is the guide to treatment methods. For instance, suppose in the informal assessment you discover that a child cannot hop on one foot. Later in treatment you are teaching this child verbs with *ing* and one of the action words you want to use is *hopping*. Referral to the initial assessment would tell the clinician that he should demonstrate and have the child use a two-foot hop as he says *hopping*. In other words, careful developmental observations will enable treatment to be planned considering the developmental level of the child so that you are doing language therapy rather than physical therapy.

Other developmental observations should provide direct guides for treatment. Informal observation of distractibility and attention span would provide the clinician with direction about whether effective treatment for this child could be conducted in a distractible environment, in a semiprivate environment, or whether the child needs to be isolated. Additionally, the clinician will have some guide as to whether the treatment room must be stripped of visual and physical materials or how many therapeutic stimuli can be presented. The attention span of the child should be a guide as to whether the first therapeutic need will be to direct the child's attention or to increase his attention span. The clinician may observe that this child works well for fifteen minutes and then is totally disinterested. This may guide the clinician to planning frequent short sessions. One may observe that with a break every fifteen or twenty minutes a child can work well for an hour. At the other end of the continuum, the clinician may note that a child can work very well for an hour. General discussions that may help a clinician identify hyperactivity in a child may be found in Crawford (1966) and Bakwin and Bakwin (1972).

The discussion of necessary or applicable developmental observations is not complete here but is rather suggestive of the type and use of observations. The clinician searching for examples of inventory forms to guide informal evaluation and the reporting of these evaluations may find the samples from Berry (1969) of case history (pp. 197-202) and communication and developmental observation forms (pp. 216-224, 232-235) useful. However, any clinician should be free and able to expand such an assessment.

Inner Language Evaluation

The term inner language is used hesitantly and for lack of a better term. Let us define inner language as the language of thought. Inner language is certainly a type of coding of oral language. Without delving into the argument of which comes first, inner language or oral language, inner language could be considered on various levels from preverbal stages through the complicated inner language of adults. Measures have not been developed to measure inner language. Certainly the complicated coding of adult inner language is most difficult to describe, let alone assess or determine its deviation.

The inner language assessment presented here is designed to partially determine if the child is realistically relating to the world, and if he has categorized things in the environment in some meaningful way. This type of informal observation seems essential for the nonverbal or essentially nonverbal child. Of course, we have no way of knowing if this type of child is using symbolic language in any form similar to our language; thus it may seem presumptive to label an evaluation of this type as an inner language assessment. Another term that has been suggested for similar evaluation is "cognitive behavior" (Chappell and Johnson, 1976).

Nevertheless, a great deal of information may be obtained by observing a child in silent play or in a situation in which he only babbles or says a few single words. One of the most practical methods is to provide a doll house, furniture, and a family of toy dolls. Observe how the child groups the furniture. Does he place furniture in room settings? A child who puts a baby in the crib and has the adults sitting at the table or in a car outside the house demonstrates a realistic organization of the world. Contrast this to the child who stacks the furniture like blocks—first the bathtub, then a chair, and then a stove. The doll house and dolls are interesting, but blocks may also be interesting tools. In one such evaluation, we observed a nonverbal child who first stacked the blocks and then unstacked them and carefully sorted them by color. Thus we could note categorization by color as well as a developmental level for stacking blocks. So we suggest that a practical method of obtaining information is to provide the child with common objects in his environment and watch what he does. Careful note taking during this period should provide a great deal of data about a child's perception of the world even if the clinician still has no method of knowing what internal language symbols the child is using.

Linguistic Competence and Performance

Linguistic competence refers to the conscious or unconscious knowledge that a speaker-listener must have in order to understand and produce the infinite number of novel sentences of a language. Competence is an abstraction. Once the clinician begins to describe the rules of a child's language then he is describing competence. The grammar of a language is the model of idealized competence. The relevant thing is the competence but competence can be measured in children only by some type of performance.

Why must we use some type of linguistic performance to measure linguistic competence? The model of competence is the rule system. Yet, a speaker may not be aware of the rules of a language per se. If a speaker is asked, he may not be able to write the rules or explain the rules, but he has internalized the knowledge. Thus we expect to try to arrive at an estimate of a speaker's competence through some type of performance. The competence-performance discussions of linguists (Chomsky, 1965, 1967; Slobin, 1971; Langacker, 1973; de Villiers and de Villiers, 1974) should provide the speech pathologist with the necessary theoretical background to understand the nature of the practical problem.

The practical problem for the speech pathologist is how to elicit a variety of linguistic performances so that the information can be compiled. Linguistic performance may be considered linguistic behavior. We would of course understand that performance might be influenced by such extralinguistic factors as memory, time, perception, situational stress, personality, and intelligence. Given these limitations, our problem is to use a variety of performances such as spontaneous speech samples, sentence repetition, elicited judgments, role playing, sentence completion, sentence formation, and any other ways one can design to discover the child's knowledge of language. We are quite aware that language is rule-governed behavior and so the next practical problem will be to describe a child's rule system. Although the rules per se are different, the need to classify the rules exists whether the rules are syntactic, phonological, semantic, or pragmatic.

In the various informal measures the clinician will want to find out the following:

1. The rules the child knows—those rules he used consistently.
2. Rules that are emerging—those rules the child uses sometimes but not all the time.
3. The rules that are restricted to child grammar—rules typically used by other children at the same language stage.
4. The rules that represent his iodiolect—rules particular to this one child.
5. The rules the child uses that are typical of adult grammar of his culture.
6. The rules a child is not using that might be expected at this stage of language development.

It should be understood that in order to ascertain number five, the clinician will have to depend on his own linguistic competence and for numbers three and six, the clinician may have to make a comparison with studies collected on a small sample of normal children. The bulk of the linguistic information has no normative data. Whether or not a small sample is representative of the language of a large population remains to be answered, but in this time of beginning language research we have to depend heavily on studies conducted on a few children.

Formal tests are not designed to derive a description of a child's competence. Although competence can probably not be completely assessed, the best description of a child's competence will be derived from a compilation of the child's linguistic performance in a variety of situations.

Spontaneous Speech Sample

A spontaneous speech sample refers to the collection of utterances that the child produces orally. These may be the egocentric speech of the young child who engages in verbalization and play with little concern for a listener or the speech of a child engaged in conversation. Spontaneous speech samples should always be tape-recorded. The analysis is made from the typed script of the tape recording of the spontaneous sample.

The clinician collecting a spontaneous sample must be cautious about the elicitation of the data. For instance if a clinician says, "What's that?" the response of the child will certainly be a noun phrase (i.e. a ball, candy, my book). Likewise if a clinician says, "What's the baby doing?" the child's response would typically be a verb phrase (i.e. crying, going nite-nite, eating dinner). In other words, a clinician must carefully watch his own language or he may skew the results of a spontaneous sample. Somehow speech clinicians seem to have a difficult time keeping their own verbalization minimal. A smile, nod of the head, or statements like "yes," "really," "tell me some more" often encourage more response from a child than a question or a long discussion. The younger the child, the less interested he will be in what the clinician says. Older children may require some minimal conversational feedback.

Some children may enjoy talking about a picture. Clinicians may find that a helpful technique is to show a picture to a child, then say something like, "Look at this picture. Sometimes it is fun to imagine that you know people in a picture. Then you can make up a story about these people. Think about it and you tell me a story about this picture." With younger children you may want to say, "Do you remember a story about the three bears and Goldilocks? Can you tell me that story?" Another effective story-telling technique reported by Melear (1974) is to have children draw their own picture and then tell about it. Story telling in its various forms seems to be a good way to elicit spontaneous speech from a child who is shy or reluctant to converse with you.

Some children seem to respond well to a telephone sample. The clinician may actually have a toy telephone available or may ask the child to imagine that he is using a phone. In this technique, the clinician tells the child, "Play like you are calling your mother. I'll tell you some things to ask her. You ask her these questions and then tell me what she says." Some questions that can be used include the following:

Ask mama what the dog is doing.
Ask mama why the boy has a bandage.
Ask mama where your tennis shoes are.
Ask mama if daddy fixed the car.
Ask mama if you can bring a friend home with you.
Ask mama how to cook soup.

Although this technique may limit the sample, it may be effective for some children. The clinician may extend the questions as far as his imagination allows and as long as the child is interested. Of course, the telephone method may be used to elicit specific structures as well as a more random spontaneous sample.

Some children will enjoy playing and conversing during play. Usually objects, dolls, and toys are most useful in this technique. While actual objects may be useful at any age, our experience tells us that the objects become more necessary the younger and/or less verbal the child is.

Sometimes it is useful to have another child converse with the child you need the sample for. However, in general this technique, while effective, is not practical because it is usually impossible to distinguish children's voices accurately on a tape recorder. Using several children talking together is probably only effective if there is a large age difference or if you are able to videotape the sample.

Asking a parent to tape the child at various times of the day may yield a good sample of a child's oral language. However, the danger with this is that parents often want the child to show off so they ask a lot of "what's this" questions, or have the children repeat after them, or have the child say nursery rhymes or count. While this is interesting, it seldom yields the data you need. If a parent is to tape record, the parent needs some instruction such as "Don't try to get Tommy to say anything. Just turn on the recorder when he is in the room with you and then talk to him as you normally would." Parents should also be cautioned not to have other siblings recording with the child.

We have discussed some of the problems of other children as elicitors of spontaneous samples but we have not mentioned the effect of the adult elicitor as a person. A recent study (Olswang and Carpenter, 1978) demonstrated that language disordered children's oral language samples showed that the quality of the language of the child was the same whether the mother or the clinician was the elicitor. The only difference was that the children used more utterances with their mothers than with the clinicians in the same time period. Insofar as the data now shows, the clinician should be confident in his ability or in the parents' ability to elicit a spontaneous language sample.

The preceding discussion of eliciting spontaneous samples provides some theoretical and practical suggestions. General guidelines for language sampling that may expand this discussion are found in Eisenson (1972), Johnson, Darley, and Spriestersbach (1963), and Longhurst (1974).

After the spontaneous language sample has been collected, the clinician should begin transcribing the tape recording. A typed transcription is recommended for clarity and ease of reading. Type each utterance on a separate line. The end of an utterance is usually clearly marked by the speaker's pause and inflection (dropping for declarative sentences and rising for questions). However, a speaker's use of pauses may be varied and Eisler (1968) provides discussion of pauses in speech. Anyone who has tried to type a language sample knows that the real problem comes when the clinician tries to ascertain whether two sentences are conjoined with *and* or *'cause* or whether the child is merely using *and* or *'cause* as starter phrases for the beginning of sentences. For these difficult decisions, the clinician must rely on intuition based on careful listening experience. The clinician will simply have to make an educated decision as to the end of an utterance.

In the typing of a spontaneous sample, great care must be taken for the accuracy of transcription. Write down exactly what the child says. For instance, if the child says "Johnny is a good boy?" you write that and *not* "Is Johnny a good boy?" In other words, do not change the child's utterance into an adult grammatical version. Be certain that you write exactly what the child said. Articulation errors are not recorded in a language sample. For instance if the child has a frontal lisp and says "Thoup ith good." you type the language utterance as "Soup is good." On the other hand, be aware of modifications of morphological inflectional endings and type them precisely as said. For instance, if a child says, "I have two shoe," that is exactly what you write.

After you have typed a transcription you need to note whether this is a representative sample. Assuming the clinician has avoided *yes/no* type questions and questions that elicit labeling or verbing, the next question will center around whether you have enough utterances. Researchers have reported using a varying number of utterances from the traditional fifty utterance sample (McCarthy, 1930) all the way to 175 utterances (Moorehead and Ingram, 1973). The outcome of this seems to be that one certainly should not take less than fifty utterances of a verbal child and the more you get the better sample you have. However, some children will not have a repertoire of fifty utterances. In this case you may need to state that you have collected thirty-minute samples or forty-five-minute samples or whatever time was spent.

After the sample has been typed, an analysis of the sample must be made. Traditionally, the words or morphemes in an utterance were counted. Although counting words gives the clinician some rough index of the child's language abilities, the objection to counting the length of an utterance is primarily two-fold: (1) Word length provides no index of the linguistic complexity of the sentence. (2) Word length is no help in planning treatment. An example of the problem of counting words is as follows: Suppose child A said, "The boy will be chasing the girl and the boy will be catching the girl." and child B said, "The boy will be chasing and catching the girl." Child A has used a fifteen-word sentence while child B has used a nine-word sentence. However the deletion of the redundant NP + modal + be (the boy will be) in the second sentence of the conjoined sentence has demonstrated a more advanced stage of language development but has created a shorter surface structure. These sentences have been used to demonstrate that the same sentence (same deep structure) with a surface length of nine words is more complicated than that sentence with a surface length of fifteen words. In reference to planning of treatment, suppose a child's longest sentences consist of four words—where will you begin in treatment? What words do you intend to add to his sentences, and where? Counting the length of the utterance is not an index to complexity or a guide to treatment. If counting words seems to be inadequate, what is done with a spontaneous sample?

One productive technique is to write a syntactic analysis of a child's sentences. Clinicians who have linguistic training may do such an analysis freestyle. Several authors (Hannah, 1977; Tyack and Gottsleben, 1974; Crystal, Fletcher, and Garman, 1977; Blackley, Musselwhite, and Rogister, 1978) have suggested guidelines for writing syntactic analyses. The clinician might want to try several of the methods in order to determine whether any of these facilitate syntactic analysis of spontaneous speech.

The type of analysis suggested by Crystal, Fletcher, and Garman (1977) is probably the most complicated but it is also quite useful. They suggest analysis in seven steps that they call scans. In scan one all sentences that cannot be analyzed are taken from the data for later consideration. The sentences that are deferred are unintelligible utterances, symbolic noises (such as sounds for cars, sirens, animals, etc.), and deviant sentences. They define deviant sentences in the very narrow linguistic sense that a sentence is deviant only when it violates basic grammatic rules such as "Dogs eating are." In their book these authors say that people using their analysis may want to modify some of the steps to suit themselves. Feeling free to demonstrate professional freedom, we might suggest a slightly different approach to scan one.

We have found that for samples from children three years and older, separating all sentences that demonstrate any modification is quite useful. The clinician would not discard these utterances but would retype on a separate sheet all modified sentences. In later scans, these sentences are analyzed just as the grammatical sentences are. We have found that it seems to facilitate our summary to see all modified sentences typed on one (or several) sheet, and all grammatical sentences in another place. When the rules are written for each sentence, all the grammatical rules will be together and easily compiled and all the modified rules will be together and easily compiled. Clinicians might follow either of these suggestions or use a method of their own.

Scan two provides an analysis of normal and abnormal response types. This enables the clinician to separate responses from initiated utterances. Part of this scan is also designed to distinguish novel utterances from imitated sentences.

Scans three and four are designed to provide an inventory of complex sentences in that one counts the connectivity (use of several sentences in one sentence), coordination, and subordination in the sentence structure. In children with disorders these scans usually do not take much time but are a useful inventory of the number of complex sentences a child has used.

Scans five and six are for the syntactic analysis of each sentence at the sentence level and at the phrase level (NP, VP). In scan seven the word structure is considered. For instance, considered in this scan are uses of such things as morphological markers of plural or past tense, verb + *ing*, auxiliary *is* (is running) versus copula *is* (John is nice), etc. Finally in scan eight one looks for any other problems not accounted for in previous scans.

Crystal, Fletcher, and Garman provide a type of summary sheet just as other authors do. We have also found it quite useful in a diagnostic summary to write out the rules a child uses grammatically and those the child modifies. However, modified sentences are most helpfully accounted for by (1) rules that indicate modifications typically expected of children this age level, (2) rules that indicate modifications typical of younger children, (3) rules that are bizarre or unusual, (4) rules that are always used versus ones that seem optional.

A problem that faces each adult analyzing a child's language sample are utterances that are extremely difficult to analyze. The practical fact is that you may have to set aside certain difficult utterances for later study. If you can analyze most of a child's utterances, do not stop because you cannot analyze a few. You will have the primary guidelines from those that can be clearly analyzed.

The clinician may need to know about research comparisons of different types of analysis of spontaneous speech (Longhurst and Schrandt, 1973) or may want to compare various methods for himself in order to see which method seems most appropriate for him to use. Comparisons have also been made between the spontaneous speech sample and the expressive section of formal tests (Prutting, Gallagher, and Mulac, 1975). Longhurst (1974) has collected a series of research studies on collection and analysis of spontaneous speech.

The spontaneous speech sample seems to be an effective method of gathering linguistic data from children. It certainly is not an end-all method because there are inherent problems. One of these problems is that performance errors might indicate a competence level below the actual competence of the person. As adult speakers, we are frequently aware of our performance errors and will correct ourselves. Children seem to rarely self correct. Thus, only by obtaining a number of examples of the same structure can we ascertain whether the sentence uttered demonstrated rule knowledge. Another problem is that in any one sample the child may not use all the structures he has knowledge of and is capable of using. The older and more verbal the child is, the more these problems are compounded. A poor spontaneous sample is of marginal value while a good spontaneous sample is invaluable as long as we realize the limitations.

Another method that may be used to expand the spontaneous sample while maintaining control of the information demonstrated is to elicit specific structures from the child.

Eliciting Specific Structures

Further assessment of syntax will probably be designed for one or both of the following reasons: To assess the child's use of a structure that did not occur in formal testing or in spontaneous speech or to assess in some depth a structure that the child has modified. The clinician's purpose is to plan treatment so time will be spent only on those structures a child should have acquired at his stage of development.

As the clinician investigates each structure under consideration, the informal measure should be designed to test samples of every possible variation of that structure and more than one example of each variation. Variations of the structure are provided throughout the discussion. One example might be if the clinician suspects the child cannot conjoin sentences with *and,* he may wish to choose a nonreduced structure such as "the mouse found the cheese and the mouse ate the cheese." Using the optional deletions, this same sentence can be changed structurally nine different ways. We can get sentences such as "the mouse found and ate the cheese," "the mouse found the cheese and ate it," etc. More than one example of a noun phrase object and subject deletion in a conjoined sentence as was used in "the mouse found and ate the cheese" can be provided by "the boy will be chasing and will be catching the girl."

One of the most accepted methods for linguists to gather data for grammar writing has been to ask an adult if various sentences were acceptable or good sentences in their language. Eliciting direct grammatical judgments from children has seemed an impossible task. An early study by Brown and Bellugi (1964, p. 135) reported what happened when a twenty-seven-month-old child was asked, "Which is right, two shoes or two shoe?" The child responded, "Pop goes the weasel." For a time following this study, authorities in children's language assumed young children could not make judgments. In 1972 Gleitman, Gleitman, and Shipley asked three two-year-old children to judge sentences as "silly" or "good." They first had the children listen to the mothers do the task and then the mothers gave the children different sentences but asked the children to tell them whether the sentences were silly or good. Silly sentences consisted of word reversals as in "Ball me the bring." or in telegraphic sentences as in "ball bring." They reported that two of the subjects scored correctly on 75 percent of the items and the third subject refused to respond. These researchers concluded that at two years of age some children have a minimal capacity to make judgments.

In studies with older children other results are appearing. Gleitman, Gleitman, and Shipley (1972) asked children five to eight years to judge sentences and de Villiers and de Villiers (1974) asked twelve-year-old children to judge sentences. In both studies the children were able to judge right and wrong at least 80 percent of the time but could not syntactically correct the sentences. De Villiers and de Villiers decided that judging grammatically was inadequate to determine rule acquisition because the children's spontaneous performance exceeded their judgment.

These studies asked children to decide right or wrong structures. Using a different approach, Willbrand (1976a) asked nine-year-olds, "Would you say 'Yesterday I writted a letter?'" etc. with a number of choices including the grammatical version. The children were quite willing to make judgments. They were also willing to select sentences adults would say and frequently selected the grammatical sentences for the adult and a modification for themselves. In an unpublished study we found that the judgments from another group of eight- and nine-year-old children about what they would say was in total agreement with their spontaneous language sample for four of the subjects and for one subject was in 85 percent agreement. Thus children seem to be accurate informants. We might then question whether it is fair to ask a child is this question right or wrong or silly—according to whose rules? The better question to ask the child seems to be "would you say. . . ?"

No doubt the younger the child is the less likely he will be willing to make judgments; however, the real problem exists in the spontaneous speech analysis of older children. Suppose that in the spontaneous speech sample the child has said, "Me and Jane have six book." and that this sentence is the only evidence of a conjoined sentence with deletions resulting in conjoined subjects (me and Jane) with the subject pronouns, and the only evidence of what should have been a regular plural (books). You might well want to expand the samples by asking the child, "Would you say, 'me and Jane are going to the store,' 'Jane and I are going to the store,' or 'Jane and me are going to the store'?" In another question you might want to ask, "Would you say 'we have six book' or 'we have six books'?" You can expand this inquiry using many different regular plurals.

While gaining grammatical judgments is still a debatable approach, it does expand the clinician's method of data collection and elicit more information about specific structures. Other methods of eliciting specific syntactic data may be used.

One efficient method of determining specific sentence structures is to have a child repeat sentences. Sentence repetition seems to assess the child's knowledge of rules on the premise that if the child has not acquired the rule, he will modify the sentence and demonstrate by his modification the rules he has acquired. However, the relationship that memory and age as well as the interest of the child have to sentence repetition has not been determined. It seems wise to warn a clinician making up sentences to remember that the sentences can be too short (therefore a child could repeat from memory as one would a digit span test) or too long. Additionally, if the child has been taught by an imitation method, such as is frequently used for hearing handicapped children or in programs of behavior modification, this method of treatment could influence repetition of sentence methods. Theoretical issues and the performances of children with language problems may be considered in more depth through research studies (Dukes and Panagos, 1973; Menyuk and Looney, 1972a, 1972b). Using a predesigned sentence repetition task, Schwartz and Daly (1978) showed that sentence repetition was an efficient method of identifying specific errors and evaluating pretherapy and posttherapy abilities. They concluded that sentence repetition could be used effectively to increase the precision of clinical assessment and treatment of language disorders.

With some care the clinician can design a sentence repetition task for a particular child. Suppose you note in the spontaneous sample several examples of omission of *be (is)* before *ing* as in "The boy running away." or "She going to school now." You may want to determine how this child will use this structure in repetition of sentences. You can ask the child to say after you, a number of sentences containing be + *ing* verbs. Bc ccrtain to include more than one sentence for each form you want to evaluate. If the child continues to omit or substitutes the *be* form in his repetition, you have pretty clear evidence that he has not acquired this rule. If the child correctly repeats the sentences several answers are possible: (1) The spontaneous speech sample demonstrated performance errors not typical of the child's performance. (2) This structure is emerging in his language but is not mastered. To clarify the answer, the clinician may need to listen to more spontaneous speech or elicit responses using other methods.

Another method that C. Chomsky (1969) used to elicit specific structures of normal children can be easily adapted to the evaluation paradigm. In this approach you use dolls or puppets and say to the child, "Have the boy ask the clown to do a somersault." Of course you design your requests to elicit the structure you are testing.

Morphology, or inflectional endings, indicating number or tense, may also need to be considered. In an investigation of normal children's acquisition of rules, Berko (1958) described a technique of eliciting knowledge of morphological rules through the use of nonsense words. For instance, she used a picture of a charming nonexistent type of creature and said to the child, "Here is a wug. Here are two of them. There are two ....." A clinician may use this technique to see if a child has a knowledge of morphological rules. However, language disordered children in our clinic have seemed to enjoy and respond to the noun plurals with nonsense words but have become confused when nonsense words were used for morphological inflections of verbs or adjectives. Even if one chooses the nonsense words, they are clinically useful only for regular markers *(s, es, ed, ing)*.

The clinician may design more direct methods of eliciting plural rules by the use of actual objects or pictures and the use of the technique of "here is a ...." and "here are two ....." If a child seems to have difficulty with plurals an assessment should include regular plurals using *s* (cats), *z* (dogs), *es* (glasses). A variety of irregular plurals that include those that change by final consonant change (wolves, calves), by mutation (mice, geese), by *en* (children, oxen), and those that do not change such as the zero morpheme plural (deer, sheep) and summation words (scissors, pants) may need to be assessed.

In addition to the sentence completion method, a direct method that provides a series of choices may be used to elicit the past tense. In this type of assessment you say to the child, "Today you are writing a letter. You did the same thing yesterday. Suppose you want to tell me about that. Would you say, 'Yesterday I wrote a letter,' 'Yesterday I writted a letter,' or 'Yesterday I wroted a letter'?" In this case the child is given the idea with three sentences but the number of choices presented lets him use his own grammar to respond. For instance, the above sample has provided the correct irregular past tense and two typical child variations (the regular past tense and the irregular stem plus the regular *ed* marker). We have found a number of children responding to this method by selecting one of these as well as by using their own form of irregular such as "Yesterday I writ a letter."

In the assessment of past tense, the first rule the child acquires is the regular *ed* marker, so these must be assessed. Irregular verbs are another problem. If you suspect a child has problems with irregular verbs you may have to consider each irregular verb. Each irregular verb may be a case unto itself. Several formal tests include *ate* and *saw* as irregular forms but these are apparently early acquired forms of the irregular verbs and are not indicative of other irregular past tense words such as *wrote* or *understood* (Willbrand, Milkovich, and Peterson, 1978).

The clinician may design many clever ways to elicit specific syntactic structures. The choice is about as variable as one's imagination. If one technique with a certain child is not eliciting the specific structure desired, then a change in method is called for. The more experience a clinician has with informal elicitation the more confident he will become of how to elicit specific data; so be willing to experiment. The worst that can happen is that you will not elicit the structure. The clinician should be certain that the child really does not use a rule rather than that the child could not demonstrate his knowledge because the method of elicitation was not productive.

The discussion thus far has concentrated on syntactic analysis.

This is in keeping with our view on the centrality of syntax. Furthermore, since more is known about syntax than other linguistic aspects of child language, it seems this may be the most fruitful area for informal evaluation. Other components of language may need to be considered as well.

Phonological Analysis

One of the informal assessments that should be made is of a child's sound system. We have defined phonology as the sounds of language. The purpose in a phonological assessment will be to determine the phonological rule system that a child is using. The need to specify the rules a child uses and to differentiate those rules that are deviant or idiosyncratic is precisely the same as in syntactic description. Of course the types of rules are different.

The language sample that the clinician will use for a phonological description may vary. In terms of an adequate sample, the one point that is clear is that the traditional articulation tests where sounds are tested in initial, medial, and final position do not provide adequate data for a phonological analysis.

The data may be collected through a spontaneous language sample or elicitation methods (see Winitz, 1975). A spontaneous sample of conversational speech is an excellent way to get a representative sample of the child's speech. Faircloth and Faircloth (1970) concluded after a research study that the spontaneous speech sample was superior to the use of isolated words. Ingram (1976) has supported the use of a spontaneous sample because he thinks that it provides a picture of the language of the child that seems missing from any other method. Some of the problems with a spontaneous sample for phonological analysis (i.e. that it may not include all the child is capable of) are similar to the problems of a spontaneous sample for syntactic analysis. However, one different and major problem in the phonological analysis is writing the transcription from a running sample; this is often complicated by the fact that many children needing a phonological analysis have basically unintelligible speech.

So other methods of specific elicitation are important. McReynolds and Engmann (1975) suggest using E. T. McDonald's (1964) *Deep Test of Articulation.* Compton (1976) has devised his own set of pictures and asks the child to name the picture. Ingram (1976) suggests that sentence completion and sentence repetition are satisfactory methods of elicitation. Ingram further expands his discussion by suggesting that a reasonable solution to gathering data is to use a combination of a variety of methods. Regardless of the method used, all of these researchers seem to agree that a sound must be tested in varying contexts, certainly in more than one word.

The types of rules written will vary. Generative phonology has provided one theory to analyze the structure of this sound system. This theory postulates a set of abstract features that are binary in nature and describe the underlying structure of sounds. An analysis of the errors on these distinctive features has proven a new and useful approach to analyzing a child's use of the phonological aspects of language. The distinctive feature approach is usually based on Chomsky and Halle's (1968) theoretical feature system. Schane (1973) has more recently written about the same theory in what seems to be a more easily understood presentation.

Researchers (Parker, 1976; Lewis, 1974; McReynolds and Huston, 1971; Pollack and Rees, 1969) have demonstrated the usefulness of the distinctive feature theory as a practical tool in the clinical setting.

Using Chomsky and Halle's distinctive feature system, McReynolds and Engmann (1975) have presented detailed guidelines for the clinician wishing to do a distinctive feature analysis. They suggest collecting a sample of each sound in varying contexts, and they say that consistent errors on ten varying contexts usually provides sufficient data. In this method, correct responses and substitution responses are analyzed. This method does not allow analysis for distortions. Each phoneme is analyzed for thirteen features. The thirteen binary (+ or −) features are vocalic, consonantal, high, back, low, anterior, coronal, round, tense, voice, continuant, nasal, and strident. For instance, the distinctive features of the /m/ sound are + consonantal, + anterior, + voice, and + nasal with all other features minus (−). The clinician will record the test phoneme, number of times of correct use, phonemes substituted, and number of occurrences and analyze these by the distinctive features. The number of omissions is recorded and finally, the number of times each feature is used correctly is recorded.

Following this analysis for each phoneme, one must make a chart for each feature. For instance, using examples from McReynolds and Engmann (1975, p. 63), an analysis sheet for continuant contrasts analyzed the phoneme in which the + continuant feature is present (i.e., f, v, θ, etc.) and in which the − continuant feature is present (i.e., p, b, t, etc.). Then the number of possible occurrences of each sound is noted, followed by the number of correct occurrences. Finally, one can figure a total number of the possible occurrences and the total of correct occurrences of the feature across all sounds. Then the percent of incorrect use is computed. The ultimate outcome is a summary of the percent of incorrect use of each feature. For instance, using examples from the summary sheet of one child (p. 99), one could note the percent of times that features are incorrect as follows:

+ vocalic	27%
− vocalic	5%
+ high	47%
− high	17%
+ low	0%
− low	9%

Of course the above example is not complete. The complete summary sheet contains the percent that is correct for each of the thirteen binary features.

The distinctive feature theory does provide one linguistic method of sound analysis, but it is like a much more traditional description of sound production in that it assumes that children acquire sounds independent of the constraints of any specific word. Other professionals such as Ingram (1976) and Compton (1976) have been quite specific about the necessity of transcribing the whole word so that one may consider the effect of the word on both correct and incorrect sound production. While it has not been definitely established that the word in which a sound appears makes the difference in production, the evidence seems to indicate that at least for some children it does. Still only through whole word transcriptions can one really analyze the individual's sound system.

Ingram (1976) suggests as narrow a transcription of each word as possible. In addition to the text and transcription of a spontaneous speech sample, he says to provide another list of each word used in alphabetical order so that the clinician can easily group at least initial sounds. They can also be listed alphabetically by final sounds as well. Examples from Ingram's (p. 65) summary of the phonological analysis of one child were the following:

Perceptual level
    Syllables: predominance of monosyllables
    Segments: the perceptually salient initial consonants are p, b, t, d, s, etc.
    Phonological processes:
        Deletion of final consonants: $C \rightarrow \emptyset \; / \_ \; \#$
        Fronting: $\begin{bmatrix} k \\ g \end{bmatrix} \rightarrow \begin{bmatrix} t \\ d \end{bmatrix}$

Organizational level
    Syllables: CV
            CVR
            CV t/d a

    Segments:
        $C_1 = p \quad t \qquad v = i \quad u$
              $b \quad d \qquad\qquad I \quad \upsilon$
                      $e \quad o$

    Phonological processes:
        Nasalization: $w \rightarrow m$ (optional)
        Lisping: $\begin{bmatrix} t \\ d \end{bmatrix} \rightarrow \theta$ (optional)

Production level:
    $C_1 = p \quad t \qquad C_2 = t/d$
          $b \quad d \qquad\qquad m$

Once again this is not an attempt to present the entire method used by Ingram but rather to give representative examples of his type of description. The symbols in the rules have been explained in Chapters 1 and 2.

Ingram (1976) and Compton (1975) demonstrate similar methods of how to keep records of reevaluations although their rule descriptions are somewhat different. A more detailed discussion of Compton's rule system was presented in Chapter 2. You may recall that he used percentages following rules to indicate how often the rule applied. Thus without discussing the rule system in detail, some examples from Compton (1976, p. 76) of the recordings of two evaluations follow:

Rule		*Reevaluation #1*
1a.	$\begin{bmatrix} p \\ t \\ k \end{bmatrix} \rightarrow \begin{bmatrix} p = \\ t = \\ k = \end{bmatrix}$	/#—optional 15%
1b.	$\begin{bmatrix} b \\ d \\ g \end{bmatrix} \rightarrow \begin{bmatrix} p \\ t \\ k \end{bmatrix}$	/#—optional 50%
3.	$[v] \rightarrow [b]$	/#—optional 80%
8a.	$\begin{bmatrix} r \\ l \end{bmatrix} \rightarrow [w]$	/#—if /r/ obligatory if /l/ optional 50%

Rule	*Reevaluation #2*
1a.	no longer present
1b.	no longer present
3. $[v] \rightarrow [b]$	#—optional 80%
8a. $[r] \rightarrow [w]$	/#—optional 90%

The clinician may need to try several different types of phonological analyses to determine which seems the most productive. Although the analysis of articulation disorders has been established for a long time, the phonological analysis of children's sound systems is relatively new. While information is now appearing, this kind of linguistic analysis is newer than the syntactic analysis. However, less well described is the category called semantic rules; this will be the topic of the next section.

Semantic Analysis

At the present time little is known about children's acquisition of semantics, so we have little to base informal assessment or the results of such assessment on. It seems apparent that we cannot assume that if a child can produce a structure that he understands it. This is probably more important as the child gets older. A current trend has been to approach language acquisition from a semantic perspective (Bloom and Lahey, 1978). Speech pathologists who seek practical application of theoretical investigations should be aware that semantic suggestions at this time are tenuous. Bloom (1970, p. 233) expressed this idea when she stated, "The study of children's language is problematical. Given the current limitations in theories of linguistics and cognition, any attempt at describing and explaining language development must be considered exploratory and tentative." Bowerman (1976) recently pointed out that the semantic classifications have varied and the results of those studies using semantic categories have conflicted. She said only further research would indicate whether semantic concepts do play a role in child language acquisition or whether semantic categories are a "convenient vocabulary" for the researcher (p. 155).

In the study of normal child language, researchers (Bloom, 1970; Brown, 1973; Schlesinger, 1971; Slobin, 1971) have presented tables of semantic categories to classify children's utterances at the two-word utterance stage based on the premise that semantic descriptions more adequately account for this stage of development. These investigators have all used adult interpretation of the children's utterances. The contention is that early utterances are interpretable by adult observers and are therefore understood. Thus adults have proceeded to design semantic categories for child language and further to classify a child's utterance into these categories.

The difficulty of the adult determining the semantic intepretation of the young child has been mentioned. Miller and McNeill (1969) citing "two boot" as a seemingly apparent example of modifier + head stated that adult "intuitions are quite compelling, but of course they could be quite wrong. The child may not have intended these sentences in the way that we interpret them" (p. 719). Anderson (1975) had the examiner and the mother independently interpret each of the eight children's two-word utterances. During weekly visits he made independent decisions about the meaning and questioned the mother about the meaning. Using Slobin's (1971) table to classify function of utterance, he found low reliability between mother and speech clinician. The agreement averaged from a low of 36 percent to a high of 68 percent. The question we might ask is just who—the person knowledgeable about children's language or the person who lives and communicates with that child—knows what the child means. Obviously, it is a moot question.

The difference of child language and the problems of adults' interpretation have been demonstrated in the study of the language of older children. Willbrand (1976a, 1976b) reported that some of the semantic differences of normal nine-year-olds were missed by adults in conversation with the child. Such sentences were syntactically appropriate and seemed semantically apparent but became ambiguous because the children interpreted the sentence in one way and the adult in another. The children proficiently used and responded to sentences that they interpreted quite differently from adults. The child's interpretation emerged only by direct questioning. The semantic differences resulted in problems in message communications that were missed by child and adult as each continued the conversation with different messages. The evidence of semantic differences elicited by direct questioning of older children makes suspect interpretations of the language of young children who cannot be direct informants.

In the case where the adult interpreter is both linguist and mother of the child, as in Bowerman's (1974, 1976) studies, we see additional problems emerging. She reported the different strategy each of her children used in approaching language acquisition. She noted that the rules for word combinations were individualistic for each child. Her data also demonstrated that many utterances over a period of time combined to provide evidence that ultimately determined the individual child's semantic categories. In addition to the problem of the adult interpreter, the following problems should be considered. We should first determine a given child's strategy for language acquisition—this strategy may not be predominately semantic categorization. If we do determine that the strategy is semantic, the language data may be insufficient to permit the adult to make semantic judgments. Certainly most diagnostic situations do not lend themselves to such extensive data. Furthermore, the problem of the individualistic categorization indicates that the use of predetermined categories with normal children is impractical. This renders current semantic tables virtually useless for analysis and suggests individual rules should be written for each child.

The problems of adult interpretation of the semantic intentions of children too young to speak for themselves seem to present evidence that current semantic analyses are research methods awaiting refinement and proof. Unproven methodology seems an unlikely candidate for practical clinical application.

Nevertheless, speech pathologists have begun to report clinical tools using semantic categories at the level of two-word utterances. McDonald and Blott (1974) devised a diagnostic strategy called "The Environmental Language Inventory" using Schlesinger's semantically based rules. They do not provide an entire test but present representative samples to demonstrate how a clinician can elicit specific structures in addition to spontaneous speech analysis.

Their method of elicitation involves linguistic and nonlinguistic cues in two procedures. In the first procedure the examiner throws a ball in the air and says, "Tell me what I'm doing." The purpose of this procedure is to elicit conversation. The second procedure is a type of sentence repetition task. In this task the examiner throws the ball in the air and says, "Say, 'Throw ball.'" They have used Schlesinger's categories but present utterances of varying complexity. Some examples of their strategy (p. 250) can be found at the top of next page.

McDonald and Blott say that they have only suggested stimuli to elicit various rules. Using this strategy the clinician may devise his own stimuli and cues to suit the level of the child being tested.

Semantics might be more clearly assessed after the child can explain for himself. C. Chomsky (1969) used a blindfolded doll and said to the child, "Show me the doll is easy to see." If the

Cued Conversation Linguistic Cues	Nonlinguistic Cues	Cued Imitation Linguistic Cues
	Agent + Action	
1. "Tell me what I am doing."	Examiner takes pen and paper and writes.	"Say 'you write' "
2. "Tell me what's happening."	Examiner shows picture of a boy swimming.	"Say 'he is swimming' "
	Action + Object	
1. "Tell me what I'm doing."	Examiner throws ball.	"Say 'throw ball' "
2. "Tell me what I did."	Examiner kicks the ball.	"Say 'kick the big ball' "
	X + Location	
1. "Tell me where it is."	Examiner puts ball on chair away from child.	"Say "ball there' "
2. "Tell me what you did."	Examiner opens bag, gestures for child to put doll in bag.	"Say 'I put doll in bag' "

child took the blindfold off the doll it was apparent this structure was not understood. This method of "show me" can easily be extended to other structures.

When a child is older a simple request such as "tell me what that means" will provide a view to the child's semantic interpretation. For instance, we heard a normal nine-year-old child say, "I can hit it four out of five times." In response to the question what does that mean, the child responded, "That means once. Four from five is one you know." The same method worked for a four-year-old who said, "A long time ago I ate an egg." In response to "when did you eat the egg?" she said, "Yesterday." But in response to "What does that mean?" she said, "It means I ate the egg for my breakfast before I comed here. That was a long time ago."

Semantic assessment should be conducted directly. However, semantic conclusions are probably more accurately completed after continuous observation of the child because the semantics will depend on the interpretation of various situations. For instance, we were working with a child who looked out of the window and said "snow"—quite appropriately labeling the white flakes. However, a few days later she insisted to her teacher that raw cotton was snow. After investigation we discovered that white powdered soap and small bits of paper were also snow. Clearly the semantic distinctions of snow were not established for her.

We have hesitantly provided these suggestions for semantic analysis because at this time any semantic approach to language disorders should be considered experimental. Speech pathologists are really hard pressed to describe a disorder when normal semantic stages have not been described, at least not beyond the two-word utterance stage. Clinicians attempting to use a semantic approach to analysis of a child's language should realize current limitations. Although the area of semantic analysis is open to speculation, pragmatic analysis is even more speculative.

Pragmatic Analysis

We defined pragmatics as the use of language in social context. In a discussion of pragmatics of children with language problems, Bates (1976) presents a series of unanswerable questions to be researched—this basically seems to be the status of research in this area at that time. However, Bates and Johnston (1977) discussed possible methods of analyzing language samples from a pragmatic perspective. For instance, in terms of conversational postulates they suggest with relevance postulates we might consider percent of time in contact, number of topics within a certain number of minutes, number of child's response turns compared to number of partner turns, and number of child's turns with topic holding trappings compared to partner's turns. They suggest that with belief postulates one might consider such behaviors on a continuum of competency from the child is an unreliable informant, to the child is a reliable informant, to the child uses sarcasm and irony.

They then suggest analysis of structural forms with pragmatic relevance such as nouns marked with indefinite and definite articles and adjectives, pronouns, relative clauses, and prenominal adjectives, use of connectives (*and, then, but,* etc.), and omission of major sentence constituents.

Another area that might be considered is speech acts, which would include frequency of use of imperatives, questions, declaratives, acknowledgements (*ok, yes, uh-huh*), and placeholders *(well, ummm).* The final category they included was sociolinguistic sensitivity, which included analysis of polite language and two kinds of conversational turn taking—responses and initiation of new topics.

We have not included these suggestions in their entirety but in a short form to give the clinician some idea of what might be an important type of assessment in the future. At the present time, work in pragmatics should be experimental. We have little evidence about normal acquisition and almost no evidence about a language disordered population.

In addition to testing phonology, syntax, and semantics in clinician devised strategy, the clinician may want to assess a child's language to see where he might place in a particular program.

Testing for Placement on Specific Programs

Some prepared programs provide tests for the clinician to use. These tests are designed for the purpose of designating a particular point at which to begin a program. One example of such a testing is the series called *Programmed Conditioning for Language Test* (Gray and Ryan, 1973). The first test of this series is a sentence repetition test and has a program score that indicates the grammatical forms or programs the child completed. The adequacy score is an indicator of the child's general syntactical ability. This form, according to the authors, is not recommended for echolalic or bilingual children. On the basis of this test, the clinician selects a specific program with which to test the child. The tests for each program are called criterion tests. Elicitation of language is a specific question. If a child scores below 80 percent on a criterion test he is not placed in that program.

Other suggestions about testing for a specific type of remediation have been provided. For instance, McDonald and Blott (1974) have suggested a guideline for assessing what base a child has if one is to begin their semantic method of teaching two-word utterances. This test is less formal than the *Monterey Test* because the clinician may expand the test.

Other programs specify where the child must be in order to begin the program but allow the clinician to develop his own method of testing the child. For instance in Willbrand's (1977) pivot grammar program, she specifies that the child should use approximately twenty-five single words meaningfully before the program is begun. The clinician must then decide how to elicit the child's use of single words.

In testing to place the child on a program, the clinician should decide initially if the child's problem warrants a particular program. If it appears that the program would suit the child's need, the next problem is to decide at what point to begin the program. Several methods of making this choice are available to the clinician: a complete assessment designed by authors of the program, a partial list of suggested assessments that the clinician must expand, and criterion to begin the program with the clinician free to design his own testing techniques. After all the initial assessments are completed, the clinician should be able to present a description of the child's problem.

Compilation of Individual Language Data

Assuming that a child has a language disorder, based on the results of formal and informal testing, the description of the results of your testing should be as explicit as possible in order to provide a guide for treatment as well as an ongoing record of the child's language. Full discussions of diagnostic reports are available elsewhere. The purpose of the following discussion is to present some guidelines for describing the language problem.

The first statement you make in the description of the problem is to say, "Tommy has a language problem." In accordance with our position, using a statement such as this means you can avoid debatable, often misused, incorrectly used, or differently used terms such as aphasia, delayed language, autism, learning disability, or language disability. Several problems exist with using such labels. One problem is that the use of such labels may mean you are "hanging a label" on a child that he will have to bear forever. He may be unable to shake the label. The second and most important point is that such a label does no good; you still must proceed to explain what you mean by the term and justify the label. In order to avoid unnecessary problems say, "...... has a language problem."

The next step is to compile a description of the problem. A problem is manifested in syntax, phonology, or semantics. Each category should be described as completely as possible. The best guide is to sequence each language component developmentally. The compilation will contain a summary of normal and deviant rule use.

Following the description of the problem, describe any accompanying behaviors. The behaviors you need to describe are those that would particularly influence treatment. You may need to describe developmental levels, attention span, distractibility, etc.

Include all evaluation methods and results. This seems obvious but while formal tests are included in most folders, clinicians frequently do not include informal assessments. Some clinicians may be embarrassed and feel that their informal assessments are too haphazard to be included. Yet this informal measure may be the best treatment guide. Furthermore, informal assessments are a continuing record of a child's changes.

Include a typed transcript of the spontaneous language sample. At the top of the sample be sure to have it labeled "Spontaneous Language Sample." Then have the child's name, age, date of the sample, stimulus materials, examiner's name, and time span of the sample (e.g. 30 minutes). In addition, include results of other informal measures—include method of elicitation, samples of elicitation, and child's responses, as well as name, age, date, and examiner's name.

The compilation of the language data is the basis for treatment. All of the measures suggested here may not be necessary for each child. In addition to what is necessary, the clinician will need to use measures that most efficiently elicit information from each child. Informal language measures require an informed, imaginative, and flexible clinician. The clinician is limited only by what the child will respond to. Use any method you can invent to obtain the necessary information.

It should be obvious that such detailed descriptive procedures may well take more than one session; the clinician must be patient and collect the data. Treatment that is initiated on little or no information may be, at best, a waste of time. Careful assessment is the best guide to effective treatment.

References

Anderson, R.: Pivot grammar: Emergence, distribution and time sampling specifications. Unpublished master's thesis, University of Utah, Salt Lake City, 1975.

Bakwin, H. and Bakwin, R. M.: *Behavior disorders in children.* Philadelphia, Pennsylvania: Saunders, 1972.

Bangs, T. E.: *Language and learning disorders of the pre-academic child.* New York: Appleton-Century-Crofts, 1968.

Bates, E.: Pragmatics and sociolinguistics in child language. In Morehead, D. M. and Morehead, A. E. (Eds.): *Normal and deficient child language.* Baltimore, Maryland: Univ Park, 1976.

Bates, E. and Johnston, J. R.: Pragmatics in normal and deficient child language. Short course at American Speech and Hearing Association Convention, Chicago: November 1977.

Berko, J.: The child's learning of English morphology. *Word, 14:*150-177, 1958.

Berry, M. F.: *Language disorders of children.* New York: Appleton-Century-Crofts, 1969.

Blackley, S. B., Musselwhite, C. R., and Rogister, S. H.: *Clinical oral language sampling.* Danville, Illinois: Interstate, 1978.

Bloom, L.: *Language development: Form and function in emerging grammars.* Cambridge, Massachusetts: MIT Pr, 1970.

Bloom, L. and Lahey, M.: *Language development and language disorders.* New York: Wiley, 1978.

Bowerman, M.: Relationships of early cognitive development to a child's early rules for word combination and semantic knowledge. Paper presented at a miniseminar for the American Speech and Hearing Association, Las Vegas, Nevada, November 1974.

Bowerman, M.: Semantic factors in the acquisition of rules for word use and sentence construction. In Morehead, D. M. and Morehead, A. E. (Eds.): *Normal and deficient child language.* Baltimore, Maryland: Univ Park, 1976.

Brown, R.: *A first language.* Cambridge, Massachusetts: Harvard U Pr, 1973.

Brown, R. and Bellugi, U.: Three processes in the child's acquisition of syntax. *Harvard Educational Review, 34:*133-151, 1964.

Chappell, G. E. and Johnson, G. A.: Evaluation of cognitive behavior in the young nonverbal child. *Language, Speech, and Hearing Services in Schools, 7:*17-27, 1976.

Chomsky, C.: *The acquisition of syntax in children from 5 to 10.* Cambridge, Massachusetts: MIT Pr, 1969.

Chomsky, N.: *Aspects of the theory of syntax.* Cambridge, Massachusetts: MIT Pr, 1965.

Chomsky, N. and Halle, M.: *The sound pattern of English.* New York: Har-Row, 1968.

Chomsky, N.: The formal nature of language. In Lenneberg, E. H. (Ed.): *Biological foundations of language.* New York: Wiley, 1967.

Compton, A. J.: Generative studies of children's phonological disorders: Clinical ramifications. In Morehead, D. M. and Morehead, A. E. (Eds.): *Normal and deficient child language.* Baltimore, Maryland: Univ Park, 1976.

Compton, A. J.: Generative studies of children's phonological disorders: A strategy of therapy. In Singh, S. (Ed.): *Measurement procedures in speech, hearing, and language.* Baltimore, Maryland: Univ Park, 1975.

Crawford, J. E.: *Children with subtle perceptual-motor difficulties.* Pittsburgh, Pennsylvania: Stanwix, 1966.

Crystal, D., Fletcher, P., and Garman, M.: *The grammatical analysis of language disability.* London: Billing and Sons, 1977.

de Villiers, J. G. and de Villiers, P. A.: Competence and performance in child language: Are children really competent to judge? *Journal of Child Language, 1:*11-22, 1974.

Dukes, P. and Panagos, J.: Repetition of comprehensible sentences by children with deviant speech. *Br J Disord Commun, 8:*139-145, 1973.

Eisenson, J.: *Aphasia in children.* New York: Har-Row, 1972.

Eisler, F. G.: *Psycholinguistic: Experiments in spontaneous speech.* New York: Acad Pr, 1968.

Emerick, L. L. and Hatten, J. T.: *Diagnosis and evaluation in speech pathology.* Englewood Cliffs, New Jersey: P-H, 1974.

Faircloth, S. R. and Faircloth, M. A.: An analysis of the articulatory behavior of a speech-defective child in connected speech and in isolated-word responses. *J Speech Hear Disord, 35:*51-61, 1970.

Gleitman, L. R., Gleitman, H., and Shipley, E.: The emergence of the child as a grammarian. *Cognition, 1:*137-163, 1972.

Gray, B. and Ryan, B.: *A language program for the nonlanguage child.* Champaign, Illinois: Res Press, 1973.

Hannah, E. P.: *Applied linguistic analysis II.* Pacific Palisades, California: Sencom Associates, 1977.

Ingram, D.: *Phonological disability in children.* London: Edward Arnold, 1976.

Johnson, W., Darley, F. L., and Spriestersbach, D. C.: *Diagnostic methods in speech pathology.* New York: Har-Row, 1963.

Knobloch, H. and Pasamanick, B. (Eds.): *Gesell and Amatruda's developmental diagnosis,* (3rd ed.). New York: Har-Row, 1974.

Langacker, R. W.: *Language and its structure,* (2nd ed.). New York: Har Brace J, 1973.

Lenneberg, E. H.: *Biological foundations of language.* New York: Wiley, 1967.

Lewis, F. C., Jr.: Distinctive feature confusions in production of and discrimination of selected consonants. *Lang Speech, 17*:60-67, 1974.

Longhurst, T. M. and Schrandt, T. A. M.: Linguistic analysis of children's speech: A comparison of four procedures. *J Speech Hear Disord, 38*:240-249, 1973.

Longhurst, T. M. (Ed.): *Linguistic analysis of children's speech.* New York: Arno, 1974.

Lundsteen, S. W.: *Children learn to communicate.* Englewood Cliffs, New Jersey: P-H, 1976.

McCarthy, D.: *Language development of the preschool child.* Minneapolis, Minnesota: U of Minn Pr, 1930.

McDonald, J. D. and Blott, J. P.: Environmental language intervention: The rationale for a diagnostic and training strategy through rules, context and generalization. *J Speech Hear Disord, 39*.244-256, 1974.

McDonald, E. T.: *A deep test of articulation.* Pittsburgh, Pennsylvania: Stanwix, 1964.

McReynolds, L. V. and Engmann, D. L.: *Distinctive feature analysis of misarticulation.* Baltimore, Maryland: Univ Park, 1975.

McReynolds, L. V. and Huston, K.: A distinctive feature analysis of children's misarticulations. *J Speech Hear Disord, 36*:155-166, 1971.

Melear, J. D.: An informal language inventory. *Elementary English, 51*:508-511, 1974.

Menyuk, P. and Looney, P. L.: A problem of language disorder—length versus structure. *J Speech Hear Res, 15*:264-279, 1972a.

Menyuk, P. and Looney, P. L.: Relationships among components of the grammar in language disorder. *J Speech Hear Res, 15*:395-406, 1972b.

Miller, G. A. and McNeill, D.: Psycholinguistics. In Aronson, E. and Lindzey, G. (Eds.): *The handbook of social psychology.* Reading, Massachusetts: A-W, 1969.

Morehead, D. M. and Ingram, D.: The development of base syntax in normal and linguistically deviant children. *J Speech Hear Res, 16*:330-352, 1973.

Olswang, L. B. and Carpenter, R. L.: Elicitor effects on the language obtained from young language-impaired children. *J Speech Hear Disord, 43*:76-88, 1978.

Parker, F.: Distinctive features in speech pathology: Phonology or phonemics. *J Speech Hear Disord, 41*:23-39, 1976.

Pollack, E. and Rees, N. S.: Disorders of articulation, some clinical applications of distinctive feature theory. *J Speech Hear Res, 12*:629-645, 1969.

Prutting, C. A., Gallagher, T. M., and Mulac, A.: The expressive portion of the NSST compared to a spontaneous language sample. *J Speech Hear Disord, 40*:40-48, 1975.

Schane, S.: *Generative phonology.* Foundations of modern linguistics series. Englewood Cliffs, New Jersey: P-H, 1973.

Schlesinger, I. M.: Production of utterances and language acquisition. In

Slobin, D. I. (Ed.): *The ontogenesis of grammar.* New York: Acad Pr, 1971.

Schwartz, A. H. and Daly, D.: Elicited imitation in language assessment: A tool for formulating and evaluating treatment programs. *J Commun Disord, 11*:25-35, 1978.

Slobin, D. I.: *Psycholinguistics.* Glenview, Illinois: Scott F, 1971.

Tyack, D. and Gottsleben, R.: *Language sampling, analysis, and training.* Palo Alto, California: Consulting Psychologists Press, 1974.

Willbrand, M. L.: Language acquisition: The continuing development from nine to ten years. In Ingemann, F. (Ed.): *Mid-American Linguistics Conference Papers.* Lawrence, Kansas: University of Kansas, 1976a.

Willbrand, M. L.: Semantic perspectives of normal nine year old children. Paper presented at American Speech and Hearing Association. Houston, Texas, November 1976b.

Willbrand, M. L., Milkovich, M., and Peterson, L.: They ate, but never drank. In Lance, D., and Gulstad, D. (Eds.): *Papers from the Mid-American Linguistics Conference.* Columbia, Missouri: University of Missouri, 1978.

Winitz, H. *From syllable to conversation.* Baltimore, Md.: Univ. Park Press, 1975.

Chapter 5

LANGUAGE INTERVENTION STRATEGIES WITH THE MINIMALLY HANDICAPPED

THIS CHAPTER WILL DEAL with selected language intervention strategies for minimally handicapped children. The term minimally handicapped has been used to differentiate some of the philosophy of remediation procedures for these children from those necessary for severely and multiply handicapped children (as considered in Chapter 6). The selection of the adjective *minimally* has been reluctantly used because in no way does the term mean these children have lesser problems or need less attention. The child without severe limitations may be the most handicapped child from the perspective that the more capable the child is, the greater is the need and expectation for his language performance to meet the normal standards. These needs and expectations will probably be expressed by the people in the environment as well as by the child himself. The child who copes with limitations, has capacity for considerable change, and is struggling to meet his personal needs and those of his environment may well be the most handicapped.

The language disordered child who is basically normal except for language acquisition, who is environmentally different, who is environmentally disadvantaged, who has minimal cerebral dysfunction, or who has a hearing loss will demonstrate a primary handicapping problem—language. Language intervention programs for these children are of extreme importance. Some of the areas discussed in the chapter on the severely handicapped, such as cognitive training, environmental enrichment, or parent training, as well as the intervention cycle, may be equally applicable to this population. The clinician planning intervention strategies should be familiar with both chapters and should understand that transference of information is necessary.

The trend in this discussion will be away from behavioral modification techniques that use operant conditioning. With rare exception these children do not need the artificially restrictive controls to elicit desired language performance. With adequate treatment these children will demonstrate language growth because they want to, or are ready to, and because they have the capacity. Thus, the emphasis in the following discussion will be on strategies for eliciting language structure from a psycholinguistic perspective. The approach discussed seems most suitable for minimally handicapped children; however, we do not mean to imply that such an approach with modifications may not be suitable for severely handicapped children.

THEORETICAL MODEL

Speech pathologists are beginning to see the need to plan treatment on the basis of a theoretical model. Recently a few authors (Miller and Yoder, 1973, 1974; Cooper, Moodley, and Reynell, 1974; MacDonald and Blott, 1974; Willbrand, 1977) have presented specific theoretical models of treatment plans. Although these theoretical bases differ considerably from each other, the important point being made is that treatment should be based on some theoretical model. We might speculate that the reason for this movement toward models is the need to be more scientific in the planning of treatment.

In a discussion of the need to use a theoretical model for research studies of language behavior, Bever (in Huxley and Ingram, 1971, p. 157) stated that "A bad model is better than no model if one insists on solving a problem." We take the position that language remediation is certainly a major attempt at problem solving in the area of language behavior and that the use of a model does seem necessary.

The exact model one choses will probably depend on acceptability and applicability. If a model is to be acceptable to the user, it stands to reason that such a model must be understood and believed by that person. The theoretical model will probably not be entirely original with the user. This seems particularly true in the area of speech pathology as we begin to incorporate the theoretical foundations proposed by linguists, psycholinguists, and sociolinguists.

For speech pathologists the model must be applicable to the

clinical setting. We would have little reason to select any theoretical model that we could not ultimately apply in a very practical way to the diagnosis, description, and treatment of language problems.

If we are going to utilize models from other disciplines, we may ultimately modify such a model. The important issue seems to be the need to base treatment on a theoretical model. What you believe is not so important as knowing what you believe and why you believe it. Know what you accept, given the current limitations of your knowledge, and what data supports this theory. This approach may mean that you will incorporate ideas from several fields or from one field, but the ultimate outcome must be a specific, describable theory. This approach also means that as knowledge increases, the theory may need to be modified.

Clinicians must begin their treatment plans based on a theory. However, in dealing with children who have problems, we must face the knowledge that the practical application of a theory may need to be modified for a specific child. In general, the approach should be consistent with the theory and should remain constant.

A PSYCHOLINGUISTIC MODEL

One type of model that seems to work for most of these children is a psycholinguistic model. As this model has been developed it has involved certain philosophies. The first theoretical assumption is that a model of normal language acquisition is the most natural method to follow. Although it has not been proven that the normal language acquisition process is most effective remedially, until evidence is presented to the contrary, normal language acquisition seems to be the most viable model. Using normal language acquisition as an intervention model involves consideration of the normal sequences of development as well as consideration of how language is acquired. It also means making some assumptions about the similarity between children with normal language and with language problems.

Another theoretical assumption is that language is rule-governed behavior. The data from studies of normal acquisition has pointed out that the sequence of rule acquisition can be specified and that child language is different from adult language. When using a model of normal language acquisition, the clinician must be familiar with what rules children should be using at various stages and the acquisition sequence of these rules, as well as what rules normal children would be expected to modify at various stages. While children involved in language treatment programs are certainly not using the rules as expected, treatment can be planned to help the children acquire the rules in a normal sequence. For instance, following normal sequence children would use single words, then two-word utterances (pivot grammar or semantic categories), and then separate verb phrases, separate noun phrases, and simple sentences. If a child with a language problem was at this level, the clinician would move the child through these stages. Knowledge of the rules of language acquisition would tell a clinician not to plan treatment initiating complete sentences immediately after the child uses his first words. At a more advanced stage, he would know not to plan treatment for embedded sentences before conjoined sentences.

In addition to the theoretical assumptions that a model of normal language acquisition provides the best treatment sequence and that this sequence can be described in terms of linguistic rules, another basic assumption is about how language is acquired. A philosophical premise of psycholinguistic theory is that children possess an innate capacity for language. They use this innate capacity to acquire language. The primary or incoming linguistic data (language used in the child's environment) is sorted and processed by each individual and the output is linguistic competence. During the process of individual acquisition, the child continuously refines his language. In other words, the child is seen as a little linguist observing and processing the language in the environment and formulating his own grammar. We assume that the children discussed in this chapter possess that same innate capacity to acquire language, but for some reason have not begun to develop this capacity in the normal predictable stages.

In such a theory, language is individually acquired or learned rather than taught. The individual will develop his own grammar in predictable sequence. Using such a theoretical foundation, the role of the clinician is to provide the data that will enable the child to utilize his innate capacity. The clinician becomes a data provider rather than a teacher in the traditional sense. As we see it, this model does not suggest a haphazard method of merely providing a lot of language stimulation, but rather a carefully planned program of selective stimulation. Nearly all of these children will have been exposed to satisfactory language stimulation in the home; it is rare to see a child who has been totally isolated from talking human beings. Thus we assume these children have been exposed to language. If these children possess the innate capacity to acquire language and if they have indeed been exposed to language but have not demonstrated normal linguistic development, then a therapeutic theory should provide some assumption about how to properly stimulate the child. The assumption of this model is that certain children may be unable to process at this developmental level the vast amount of primary linguistic data that most children cope with, and, therefore, the primary data needs to be simplified for these children.

The simplification of data requires that the clinician select the structures the child needs to acquire and restricts stimulation to repeated examples of that structure. For instance, if the child is first learning single words, then the clinician might use objects or pictures and limit the clinician's verbalizations to only the single words the child needs to acquire. Thus, a clinician might decide to expose a child to only five new words at a time and in the first session would have five objects in the room (e.g. a ball, a cookie, a teddy bear, juice, and a book). The clinician would meaningfully manipulate each object but would only say "ball," "book," "cookie," etc.

At a more advanced level an example of stimulation for the pronoun *I* might be to begin by using first names of the clinician and the child. For instance, "Jane wants the pickle." or "Tommy has the pickle." After the child becomes accustomed to the use of first names the clinician can say, "Now there is another way to say this. We can say, 'I want the pickle.' 'I like pickles.' etc." This simple movement from deep structure to surface structure seems to be much more efficient than saying to the child, "Don't say 'me,' say 'I.' " It is difficult to tell a child that *me* is wrong because *me* is, of course, grammatical in the object position. Instead of a great deal of correction and explanation, the idea is to provide repeated modeling of the structure to be learned. Regardless of the level of structure, the purpose of the clinician is to provide as much data as possible so the child can process the rule. When the child is ready to experiment by using the language he hears, he will begin to do so.

Another integral part of the proposed model is not to demand that the child respond. Demanding that a child repeat just what the clinician has said or respond exactly as directed restricts the process of linguistic acquisition. The clinician wants the child to respond when he perceives the desired structure sufficiently to produce his own sentences. The ideal result is for the child to utter a novel sentence (different from any the clinician has used) using the same rule. For example, suppose a clinician was trying to elicit subjectless verb phrases; he might design a treatment session with a washing activity. He could stimulate with a number of utterances, such as, "wash the cup," "wash the spoon," "wash the baby," etc. The child might respond by repeating any of the activities and using some of the same verb phrases (e.g. "wash the cup") or the child might pick a new object to wash saying "wash the frog." While this utterance is novel, the child might present an even more novel utterance by saying "dry the cup." All of these responses would have been said because the child had processed the rule and was ready to use it and all would be acceptable because the goal of the session was to elicit verb phrases.

In such a model, how does the child know when the response he has made is appropriate? Acknowledging desired clinical responses is necessary but should be as much in keeping with a model of normal language acquisition as possible. Thus we have found that a smile, a touch, a nod of the head, and the word *good* seem to indicate that a response was what was desired.

The psycholinguistic model proposed here is based on the following theoretical assumptions: a model of normal language acquisition should be the basis for a therapeutic model, language is rule-governed behavior, children with normal and disordered language possess an innate capacity to acquire language, the purpose of the environment—both normal and clinical—is to provide primary data, and the child will individually acquire language given adequate stimulation. Some practical theoretical adjuncts include suggestions of limiting the verbal input, using a variety of utterances based on one rule, making no demands or pressures on the child to use certain language, and using a limited and natural reward for desired responses. The model proposed here is the authors' suggestion of a psycholinguistic theoretical model; it is not the only psycholinguistic model and is presented as a description of one strategy of intervention.

Clinicians wanting to develop a similar model may find the discussions of the nature of language acquisition by Chomsky (1965, 1968) and Lenneberg (1967) and of social learning theory by Bandura (1971) useful. A clinician should feel free to develop his own theoretical model for intervention, remembering that the important thing is to know what you believe and why you believe it. With that foundation, a clinician is ready to develop a theoretical model for intervention strategies.

Intervention Strategies

Intervention strategies utilizing psycholinguistic approaches are just beginning to appear. Some of the approaches have clearly stated their theoretical basis but most have not. The purpose of this section is to present some of the psycholinguistic approaches available whether or not they are accompanied by theoretical discussions. Some of the methods have been designed for specific groups of children but have a potential broad range of application. For instance, some intervention strategies using a psycholinguistic approach have been designed for severely handicapped children and use behavior modification techniques. In keeping with our previous premises, we assume that clinicians working with minimally handicapped children would know that behavior modification and/or imitation tasks are usually not necessary for these children. The approaches can be modified to suit the children with whom they are to be used. The emphasis in this section will be on clinical methods designed to help children utilize grammatical rules. Leonard (1973) has provided a discussion of the application of the idea of rule learning to the treatment of children with language problems. The methods discussed in this chapter are not the only ones available but are representative of the resources a clinician may utilize. While the clinician may utilize an established approach, the best treatment plan is one that is written or adapted to suit the needs of an individual child.

Early Intervention Strategies

Among the psycholinguistic approaches available, a trend toward early intervention strategies can be observed. In the past, intervention methods have been presented for older children and most available programs have been designed for children identified as mentally retarded, emotionally disturbed, or with other severe problems. It may have been that speech pathologists were primarily seeing children who had severe handicaps or other children after they reached school age. Speech pathologists are now seeing more and more children at young ages with minimal handicaps who have not begun to talk at the expected age or who have limited use of language. It does not stand to reason that minimally handicapped children are now demonstrating problems at an early age when they did not do so in the past, nor is it reasonable to assume that more children have early language problems than before.

There are several plausible explanations for the current interest in early intervention for children with minimal problems. One group of explanations centers around increasing public and professional awareness of problems in the early years and the effectiveness of early training. The influx of nursery schools, preschools, and Head Start programs has helped create awareness. Parents have become more informed and aware of the possibility of early education, as well as more attentive to preventive medicine in early childhood years. This awareness has probably meant that more children are brought or referred to speech clinicians than ever before. Another reason for the increasing interest in early intervention centers around changes in the speech therapy profession. This is a maturing profession with increased educational requirements, licensing and certification requirements, and members and has doubtlessly made its presence known. An important influence is the spread of information about children's language development since the late 1950s. While children's language development is still not fully understood, the growth of knowledge about language acquisition is startling. The most extensively researched area is early language acquisition. It stands to reason that professionals who believe that remediation of language problems should follow the model of normal development would begin to develop treatment programs for this early stage about which most is known.

Another possible reason for the early intervention programs is the knowledge that when children have minimal problems, early remediation may avoid or reduce the development of a much more severe problem. A language problem allowed to go unattended will build on itself. Clinicians must recognize, however, that some children will naturally develop language a little later than others and will still be within a normal range. Some families report a history of late onset of language, but if a child is a year or more delayed in language development, the need for remediation is apparent.

The theoretical bases of the early intervention strategies are as varied as the methods they employ. The following is a discussion of some psycholinguistic intervention strategies at early language development stages and not a debate of the relative merits of the theoretical model or the methods employed.

Hutchinson (1972) reported the results of clinically initiating first words. He selected single words to be taught to children on the basis of semantics, phonology, and appearance on the lips. He used nouns, verbs, and adjectives relevant to the child's needs. The first words the children established clinically were *that, that one, call, it,* and *there.*

Holland (1975) discussed the development of a core lexicon in the clinical setting. In teaching single words it is important for the clinician to remember that one-word utterances are primarily nouns, and the words taught a child need to have real-world application. The words the child learns clinically need to represent the child's wants, feelings, and environment. Holland cautions that the core lexicon developed must provide words that can be also used at the two-word utterance level, the next stage of development.

Lahey and Bloom (1977) suggested that in selecting single words to teach the clinician should consider whether or not the concept of the word can be illustrated in nonlinguistic context. They suggested using nouns to refer to objects but also including some verbs, adjectives, and prepositions. They stressed that usefulness of the vocabulary is important. For example, adjectives such as *big* or *dirty* are more useful to most children than adjectives such as *orange* or *round*. Lahey and Bloom also emphasize the acquisition of certain words. For instance, they say that *sad* or *hungry* are late developing words, as are words such as *yes* and *you*, and such words should be excluded, on basis of form and content interaction, from the first lexicon intervention strategies.

A number of intervention strategies have appeared for the two-word utterance level. Willbrand (1977) proposed a therapeutic plan for initiating two-word utterances based on pivot grammar and the principle of activating the child's innate capacity. The clinician selects pivots based on studies of normal development and models these pivots for the child one at a time in combination with open class words the child has previously established. The clinician, using modeling and expansion techniques, works with only the selected pivot and open class words. In an early modeling session, the clinician says, "see baby," "see rope," "see ball," "see cookie," "see juice," and so on. In expansion, if the child says "cookie," the clinician says "see cookie." Pivots are initiated one at a time. The child is not required or demanded to respond. The child responds as he is ready to use the language spontaneously. As soon as one pivot is initiated (indicated by child's spontaneous use ten times) another pivot is introduced. As more pivots are established, the language of the clinician might consist of a variety of pivot and open class words. The clinician might say, "see bubble," "bubble up," "bubble all gone." The pivot class remains small and a variety of open class words are used.

MacDonald and Blott (1974) devised an early intervention strategy based on Schlesinger's (1971) semantic rules (i.e. agent + action, action + object, X + location). Their method utilizes simultaneous imitation and conversation. If the clinician wants to establish the use of action + object, the clinician might throw a ball and say to the child, "Say, 'throw ball.'" and again throw the ball and say, "Tell me what I'm doing." Structural play activities in which the child is required to use the language rules established follows the imitation and conversation training. This method of treatment has been expanded into a parent treatment program (MacDonald, et al., 1974).

Miller and Yoder (1973, 1974) also proposed a remediation program for one-word and two-word utterances based on semantic categories. They use categories such as recurrence, nonexistence, rejection, etc. They propose selecting a single semantic function at a time. The selection of the semantic function depends on a relationship the child has experienced in his environment and of which the child demonstrates a cognitive-perceptual awareness. For example, if a clinician wanted to teach recurrence *more* + substantive word at the two-word level, he would follow specific therapy steps: (1) Expose the child to the experience (give a glass of milk and a moment later clinician says, "more milk"). (2) Child indicates comprehension (child looks for another glass, hearing "more milk"). (3) Clinician pairs linguistic marker with experience and asks child to imitate (child must imitate "more milk" in order to receive). (4) Clinician fades imitation and introduces spontaneous response with some semantic relationship (more cookies, more book, etc.). (5) Clinician systematically reduces modeling and imitation in order to determine spontaneous use on part of the child. Miller and Yoder state that working on only one function at the beginning leads to faster acquisition. After the first function is mastered in context, other functions can be introduced at a more advanced language development stage.

A few strategies have been suggested for helping children initiate beginning sentences. Bricker, Dennison, and Bricker (1976) suggest a model to teach children: agent + action + object sentences. Their program utilizes the following steps: attending skills, imitation, function use, comprehension, and production.

All of these strategies have been directed toward initiating language in children from first words to first sentences. Others have suggested treatment for these earliest stages of language development, but have included it as part of a series leading to more advanced language development remediation. Early intervention implies remediation as soon as a problem is identified in the preschool years. This, of course, may mean that treatment could begin at the simple sentence or transformational level as well as at the single word level. Language treatment strategies that extend beyond the simple sentence level are discussed in the following section.

Intervention Strategies Beyond Early Language

Some intervention strategies have been presented to cover varying stages of language acquisition. Gottsleben, Tyack, and Buschini (1974) discussed sample cases of treatment for early sentences and for regular plural forms. They report the results of the treatment program in terms of increase in percentages. The idea of noting language improvement in percentages may be useful to speech clinicians in the public schools who must now write IEPs (individualized education plans) for children using percentage figures.

Hatten, Gorman, and Lent (1973) and Gray and Ryan (1977) suggest methods of teaching linguistic structures beginning with single words, progressing through simple sentences, and ultimately eliciting much more advanced structures such as interrogatives, conjunctions, negatives, and verb tenses. Each program is specifically planned and the criteria to be achieved for each objective is established. The Hatten, Gorman, and Lent program uses objectives such as: "The child will produce ten three-word phrases consisting of the possessive 'my' plus the adjective 'dirty' followed by each of ten core nouns elicited by the stimulus pictures with 90 percent accuracy in the clinical setting" (p. 13).

They then follow the stated objective with one sample activity and list possible responses to be obtained. A clinician using this program is free to expand the activities and methods of elicitation. The child may make a variety of acceptable responses.

The Gray and Ryan procedure is much more structured with each program step specified. Each step and criterion is based on a stimulus-response-reinforcement system with prompts gradually faded out.

Stremel and Waryas (1974) have proposed a method of language training that progresses from simple sentences to complex sentences. Three major programs—early language training, early-intermediate language training, and late-intermediate language training—are presented in sequential steps. The sequential progression in the late-intermediate language training (the highest level) is as follows: The entry behaviors required are 90 percent accuracy of the linguistic structures in the previous or early-intermediate language training program. If these criteria are met, the child learns the following structures in sequence: interrogative reversals, conjunction *and,* regular plurals, noun and verb agreement, verb tense markers, relative clauses, and embedded sentences. Each step is taught by following a sequence of specified conditions that proceed through the general areas of comprehension, imitation, echoic stimuli, generalization, and acquisition.

Lee, Koenigsknecht, and Mulhern (1975) propose a story-telling technique to elicit a variety of grammatical structures from a child depending on the child's need. Each story has four or five grammatical targets. The clinician reads a few lines of a story and then asks the child questions to elicit the target responses. The program is not rigidly administered and the clinician may repeat from the story, as well as use a variety of prompts to elicit the desired responses. The focal points are the interaction of the clinician and the child and the development of the specific structures. The child is encouraged to formulate his own language rather than to imitate the clinician. Wallace and McLoughlin (1975) present a general approach to improve grammar. Children are taught basic sentences and transformations. Fry (1972) presents a therapy program to initiate the personal pronoun *I.*

Some of the programs described have been designed for different types of children including the basically normal child with language problems, the child with a learning disability, and the child described as mentally retarded. Other approaches have not specified a particular group of children. Some of the approaches follow a consistent psycholinguistic approach, while others combine behavioristic and psycholinguistic methods. Most of the behavioristic methods were designed for severely handicapped children, i.e. mentally retarded.

Consistent with the view previously presented in the chapter, few children with minimal handicaps need extreme behaviorist treatment in order to learn language. However, the psycholinguistic approaches presented here could easily be modified by excluding the behavioristic techniques. There may be occasions when the clinician is convinced that the therapy strategies are not being effective. In this case, he may wish to employ imitation and/or more rigorously structured procedures. However, we have seen children in our clinic who did not seem to respond to the psycholinguistic approach described as the basic theoretical premise of this chapter. They remained seemingly unresponsive for as long as four months and then began to respond quite suddenly. The clinician must be cautious about assuming that an approach does not work. A nondemanding approach such as the one we have recommended may take longer to initiate verbalization, but the ultimate outcome will be spontaneous and novel language use. A more demanding approach is certainly less natural and may be less efficient in terms of generalization.

In addition to published methods of treatment, some commercial materials designed to elicit linguistic structures are available. Representative programs and materials are found at each language level.

The *Ready, Set, Go-Talk To Me* program (Horstmeier, MacDonald, and Gillette, 1975) is a parent or teacher program based on the environmental language programs of MacDonald and Blott (1974) and MacDonald et al. (1974) discussed earlier in this chapter. These materials are designed so they can be used by parents or teachers if speech or language clinicians are not available. This program begins with attention gaining, motor imitation, and receptive skills of identifying and understanding single words. The final step is two-word combinations. The procedures at each level include what the adult should do (i.e. push the car) and what the adult should say (i.e. "What did I do?"). At each step appropriate and inappropriate responses are shown with instructions about how to proceed. For instance, if in the example given the child says "push car," the adult is instructed to give praise and go on to the next item.

The *Motivation and Learning Centered Training Programs for Language Delayed Children* (Mecham, 1974) presents a program and materials for use by speech and language clinicians that covers developmental stages from a prelinguistic level to transformations. This developmental sequence is followed: gestures, nouns, verbs, two-word, three-word, four-word, and five-word sentences, verb inflections, adjectival and adverbial modifiers, and negative and passive constructions. At all levels the teaching sequence is imitation, delayed imitation, and spontaneous use.

Two different sets of materials are designed to provide teaching aids for syntactic structures that are frequently modified by children with language problems at the simple sentence and more advanced levels. *The Developmental Syntax Program* (Coughran and Liles, 1975) is designed for remediation of articles, personal and possessive pronouns, adjectives, *be* verb, *have* verb, regular and irregular past tenses, and plurals. This program uses some traditional articulation techniques in that it has three phases of ear training, production, and generalization to varying contexts. Although the child is taught to recognize correct and incorrect syntactic structures, an important aspect of this program is that the clinician must not verbally correct any error made by the child. The plan is short and the authors suggest never administering it for more than seven and one-half minutes in any one session.

The other program designed to improve various sentence types is the *Fokes Sentence Builder* (Fokes, 1978). This program is much less structured than the other commercial material discussed here. It is an adaptable technique for eliciting sentences and allows the clinician to be innovative. The materials provided can be utilized for an individual child at whatever level the child needs. This program provides the clinician with a folding mat for the building of sentences. Sentences are "built" by seriating cards that use words for sentence elements. The cards have pictures of people, objects, and animals, transitive and intransitive verbs, and adjective concepts, as well as pictures showing position or location, manner (i.e. slowly), and temporal concepts (i.e. seasons of the year or time of day). In addition, word cards have printed on them possessive pronouns and other grammatical elements that cannot be pictured, such as *the, is, did,* etc. This is one method of helping children formulate their own sentences and techniques to elicit past, present, and future tenses; articles, auxiliary verbs, plural nouns, pronouns, and verb forms are included. The author suggests that clinicians make their own cards to expand each category and to fit the needs of an individual child. Clinicians who prefer to do their own planning and who like to have a basic set of materials that are easily augmented will probably be pleased with this less structured program.

Other commercially available programs amd materials may be purchased. These specific ones have been presented here in order to indicate types of packaged materials available to elicit specific syntactic or semantic structures.

Any of the previously mentioned programs (commercial or research) or materials may be adapted to children with various problems. The planning of intervention strategies depends on the theoretical foundation and elicitation of specific linguistic structures based upon the individual needs of each child. Intervention strategies must include knowledge of the special problems accompanying some of these children.

Special Therapeutic Considerations

Some children with minimal handicaps have special accompanying problems that a speech clinician will need to keep in mind as strategies for intervention are planned. These problems will affect treatment but not the general philosophy about language acquisition or the structure of language.

During early intervention with children who are nonverbal, using single words, or beginning two-word combinations, the clinician should strive to have materials and sessions concretely represent the real world. For example, the use of actual objects and the appropriate manipulation of these objects will probably have much more meaning for children at this stage than pictures. If a clinician tries to elicit the word *milk* from a child by using a picture, it would be difficult to determine if the child thought that she was labeling the glass or the liquid in it. Likewise it is difficult to help the child know that milk looks, tastes, etc. a certain way that is different from water, juice or any other liquid. In a similar manner to teach *ball* or *see ball* or *throw ball* without the child actually being able to feel and manipulate the object seems unreasonable. Pictures are easier for clinicians to carry about, but the purpose of treatment is to help the child acquire language for communication. The goal must be application to the real world rather than a conditioned response to a picture. We cannot flash pictures at a child and then expect him to respond in every day situations. This does not imply that pictures may not be useful in more advanced stages. Throughout this book we have emphasized that the words, phrases, or sentences a child learns should fit that child's communication needs. Many young children are delighted with bubbles that can be blown from a prepared liquid. It becomes a fairly easy task to elicit *see bubble, bubble up, bubble down* when the child can observe and participate in the action. Eliciting a verb phrase such as *wash cup, wash baby* becomes a pleasant task if the child can have a pan of water and actually wash the various objects. Extra care in early intervention to determine that the child has seen, manipulated, felt, tasted, or experienced the language she is using provides rewarding experiences for both child and clinician.

Children with minimal cerebral dysfunction or a learning disability may be distractible and/or have short attention spans. A clinician working with a distractible child will want to take extra precautions in setting up the physical environment of the treatment sessions as well as in planning intervention. The treatment room should be stripped of visually distracting materials such as pictures or posters on the wall. The clinician should consider personal attire and avoid distracting scarfs, jewelry, and brightly patterned materials. The physical environment should also be controlled for sound distractions. These children will find it more difficult than other children to ignore extraneous environmental noises. A frequent problem in the public schools is trying to conduct therapy while a group of children are at recess just outside the room where you are working. While this situation may be unavoidable, it should be possible to not schedule a distractible child for treatment during that time.

In addition to taking extra care with the environment, the clinician should guard against exposing the child to too many treatment materials at one time. Treatment will have the greatest chance of being successful when the only visible material is the one set necessary for a particular section of the session. For instance, we observed a child who became so distracted because the clinician left the flannel board with the figures on it on the table in a corner that he quit responding to the treatment. The child had been moved to another location in the room but the previously used material was still clearly visible and very distracting to the child.

Another element to be considered is the timing of the sessions. If the child has a short attention span, the clinician should plan sessions within the limits of the attention span. Attention span may be increased by planning short breaks and returning to work. With extra care taken to plan the environment and time of the session, children with cerebral dysfunction can be encouraged to produce to their maximum capability.

The culturally disadvantaged child may need to have more environmental experiences in order to use language effectively; unlike the other groups, these children may be from poor families or they may have had little experience with the world for other reasons. It may be difficult to believe but there are still children who have never been to a grocery store, seen an electric or gas stove, or seen any animals other than domestic ones.

Traditionally, attempts at language remediation focused on providing a variety of experiences for children and talking about them as well as stimulating the child to talk. In general, this approach to language remediation is not specific enough to elicit desired linguistic structures. However, if a child is truly culturally disadvantaged, the speech clinician may need to provide environmentally enriching activities in addition to those activities provided by preschools, Head Start programs, or classrooms. The clinician may also need to help teachers plan activities that will help these children have experiences, learn new vocabulary, communicate with adults, and learn to solve problems. The clinician should be aware that in any treatment session the child may not know the concept behind the language the clinician is trying to elicit.

Culturally disadvantaged children will respond better to concrete rather than abstract language use. The use of language with real objects and situations will be the more effective teaching device. The speech clinician will, of course, need to teach the structure of the language. Some remedial programs (Bereiter and Englemann, 1966; Hart and Risley, 1968; Manuchin and Biber, 1968; Reynolds and Risley, 1968; Lavatelli, 1971) have provided structured and unstructured programs for language remediation for culturally disadvantaged children. One of the problems with programs for the disadvantaged is that they are often presented for environmentally different children.

The problem of the environmentally different child is currently being approached much differently than in the past. Early approaches such as Bereiter and Englemann (1966) suggested telling the child his language was wrong or he had made an error. The current approach is to tell the child that the language is different. This shift in theoretical viewpoint is well known and has influenced the language training methods for these children. Within this perspective an educational debate still rages. In general, everyone seems to agree that children need to acquire and be able to appropriately use standard American English in order to be educated in the public schools as well as to gain social and economic advantages as adults. The debate is over how far the acquisition of standard American English should go. One opinion is that the children must learn standard American English to replace any other dialect or language they are using. Another view is that the children should learn standard American English as a second language but maintain their initial language patterns. Given this approach, the child would become bilingual and would be able to use the language of the group with whom he needed to communicate. The proponents of this way of thinking point out that the person who gives up his native communication system will no longer be accepted by the other members of his racial or ethnic community. For example, a black person who returns to a black ghetto or black neighborhood speaking standard American English will not be accepted as a viable member of that group. Advocates of this perspective strongly recommend that the person maintain both languages in order to communicate and be a part of a given community. A discussion elaborating these views may be found in Stoller (1975).

Speech clinicians may well question their role in the treatment of language difference. Of course, any child with a difference who also has a disorder should be treated for the disorder. The question becomes, is it the speech and language clinician's job to teach standard American English for children speaking a different language or dialect? We support the position of Williams (Williams and Wolfrom, 1977) who felt that when a person wants to change his language it is the speech pathologist's obligation to help him do so provided that the pathologist knows the rules and lexicon of the other language. In other words, remediation for language differences should be offered by the speech pathologist but the decision to partake of such training should be made by the person speaking the other language or dialect. Some specific guides to planning such a program may be found in Hagen and Hallahan (1970), Bentley and Crawford (1973), and Williams and Wolfram (1977).

Children with a hearing handicap also present special remediation problems. For some time, the need for early amplification has been known. Along with the need for early amplification, a great deal of stress was placed on auditory training in the early years.

The speech clinician working with hearing handicapped children will need to be familiar with methods of ascertaining whether or not the child's hearing aid is turned on and whether or not the aid is functioning. While the speech clinician does not fit the aid, he still has a need to know if an aid is operating. (For information on the operation and maintenance of hearing aids, see Pollack and Downs, 1964 and Downs, 1971.) In the early stages of treatment, the speech clinician may need to teach the child to locate, identify, and discriminate sound (see Pollack, 1970).

An additional problem to be aware of when dealing with hearing handicapped children is that these children may be environmentally disadvantaged. The greater the hearing loss, the greater the chance is that the people in the child's environment will have decreased their linguistic input to the child. Thus, the possibility exists that a hearing handicapped child may not have had the opportunity to talk about a broad range of events, let alone experience a broad range of stimuli. The clinician needs to be aware that planning treatment for the hearing handicapped child may necessitate using some of the techniques used for the environmentally disadvantaged, such as providing experiences and general language stimulation. Of course, these children need to learn specific language structure as well. Treatment methods need to provide a combination of approaches. The primary problem is to help the child acquire language. Surprisingly little stress has been placed on intervention strategies in early language training for these children. Since receiving and expressing of oral language is a major problem for these children, it is safe to assume that given current knowledge about language acquisition, more and more attention will be given to early intervention language programs for these children.

A review of language development programs has been provided in Dale (1974). While these programs may be helpful, the application of psycholinguistic principles to language training for hearing handicapped children is surprisingly absent. A few researchers have discussed the application of psycholinguistic constructs in training the hearing impaired (Streng, Kretschmer, and Kretschmer, 1978; Feldman, 1970; Moores, 1970). The newest information emphasizes a structural description and sequencing of the language. For the most part, language programs for hearing handicapped children await new methodology based on current linguistic knowledge.

The clinician who wants to design his own psycholinguistic treatment plan for a hearing impaired child may find the book by Russell, Quigley, and Power (1976) a useful guide to understanding the linguistic structure of deaf children. Information on writing goals for language structure and the grammar levels provided in Streng, Kretschmer, and Kretschmer (1978) may also supply valuable guidelines.

SUMMARY

This chapter has presented a psycholinguistic theoretical model as a basis for intervention strategies with minimally handicapped children. This model was based on the supposition that these children possess an innate capacity for language and that the role of the clinician is to provide the primary linguistic data that will enable the child to establish his linguistic rule system. The specific methods of intervention presented have all had the purpose of initiating linguistic rules. The model described here is specific but intervention methods represent a broad range of techniques and theoretical assumptions. The clinician referring to the programs will note many diverse assumptions are presented, such as "children with language disorders possess an innate capacity to develop language" (Willbrand, 1977) and children with language disorders are a "walking refutation of the idea of innate natural language development" (Gray and Ryan, 1977, p. 5). These widely different assumptions may be the result of a matter of difference of opinion or may be a matter of the difference in the type of child the program was developed for.

While we would maintain that the theoretical position presented in this book is a sound foundation for the treatment of children with minimal problems, the clinician should read the various theories and then decide for himself what theory seems the most plausible.

Because of the varying theoretical assumptions, the intervention techniques differ considerably but they have several factors in common. All intervention strategies are designed to elicit specific linguistic responses which are based on linguistic rules. In each approach, the linguistic input from the clinician is limited to utterances that elicit specific rule-oriented responses from the children being treated. Clinicians treating children with language disorders should read various strategies and design their own plans. The published research studies have reported success with very different techniques. The strategies presented here should be perceived as strategies and not as required programs. The best treatment plan for any child with a language disorder incorporates theory, techniques, and specific structures to be elicited that are chosen specifically for a particular child and clinician.

References

Bandura, A. (Ed.): *Psychological modeling: Conflicting theories.* New York: Aldine, 1971.

Bentley, R. H. and Crawford, S. D. (Eds.): *Black language reader.* Glenview, Illinois: Scott F, 1973.

Bereiter, C. and Englemann, S.: *Teaching disadvantaged children in the preschool.* Englewood Cliffs, New Jersey: P-H, 1966.

Bricker, D., Dennison, L., and Bricker, W.: *A language intervention program for developmentally young children.* MCCD Monograph, Series No. 1, 1976.

Chomsky, N.: *Language and mind*. New York: Har Brace J, 1968.

Chomsky, N.: *Aspects of the theory of syntax*. Cambridge, Massachusetts: MIT Pr, 1965.

Cooper, J., Moodley, M., and Reynell, J.: Intervention programmes for preschool children with delayed speech development. *Br J Disord Commun, 9*:81-91, 1974.

Coughran, L. and Liles, B.: *Developmental syntax program*. Austin, Texas: Learning Concepts, 1975.

Dale, D.: *Language development in deaf and partially hearing children*. Springfield: Thomas, 1974.

Downs, M. P.: Maintaining children's hearing aids. *MAICO Audiological Library Series*, vol. 10, report 1, 1971.

Feldman, D. M.: Linguistics as a basic science in the habilitation of the hearing impaired. In Berg, F. S. and Fletcher, S. G. (Eds.); *The Hard of Hearing Child*. New York: Grune, 1970.

Fry, W. H.: The challenge of personal pronouns. *Journal of Learning Disability. 2*:299-305, 1972.

Fokes, J.: *Fokes sentence builder*. Boston, Massachusetts: NYT Teaching Resources Cooperation, 1978.

Gottsleben, R. H., Tyack, D., and Buschini, G.: Three case studies in language training: Applied linguistics. *J Speech Hear Disord, 39*:213-224, 1974.

Gray, B. and Ryan, B.: *A language program for the nonlanguage child*. Champaign, Illinois: Res Press, 1977.

Hagen, J. W. and Hallahan, D. P.: Language training program for preschool migrant children. *Exceptional Children, 37*:606-607, 1970.

Hart, B. and Risley, T.: Establishing use of descriptive adjectives in the spontaneous speech of disadvantaged preschool children. *J Appl Beh Anal, 1*: 109-120, 1968.

Hatten, J., Goman, T., and Lent, C.: *Emerging language*. Westlake Village, California: Learning Business, 1973.

Holland, A.: Language therapy for children: Some thought on context and content. *J Speech Hear Disord, 40*:514-523, 1975.

Horstmeier, D., MacDonald, J., and Gillette, Y.: *Ready, set, go—talk to me*. Columbus, Ohio: Ohio State University, The Nisonger Center, 1975.

Hutchinson, M. D. F.: An experiment in applying linguistics to speech therapy. *Br J Disord Commun, 7*:49-53, 1972.

Huxley, R. and Ingram, E. (Eds.): *Language acquisition: Models and methods*. New York: Acad Pr, 1971.

Lahey, M. and Bloom, L.: Planning a first lexicon: Which words to teach first. *J Speech Hear Disord, 42*:340-350, 1977.

Lavatelli, C.: *Language training in early childhood education*. Urbana, Illinois: U of Ill Pr, 1971.

Lee, L., Koenigsknecht, R., and Mulhern, S.: *Interaction language development teaching*. Evanston, Illinois: Northwestern U Pr, 1975.

Lenneberg, E. H.: *Biological foundations of language.* New York: Willey, 1967.

Leonard, L.: Teaching by the rules. *J Speech Hear Disord, 38*:174-183, 1973.

MacDonald, J. D. and Blott, J. P.: Environmental language intervention: The rationale for a diagnostic and training strategy through rules, context, and generalization. *J Speech Hear Disord, 39*:244-256, 1974.

MacDonald, J. D., Blott, J. P., Gordon, K., Spiegel, B., and Hartmann, M.: An experimental parent assisted treatment program for preschool language delayed children. *J Speech Hear Disord, 39*:395-415, 1974.

Mecham, M. J.: *Motivation and learning centered training programs for language delayed children.* Salt Lake City: Word-making Productions, 1974.

Miller, J. and Yoder, D.: An ontogenetic language teaching strategy for retarded children. Paper presented at NICHD Conference on Language Intervention with the Mentally Retarded, Wisconsin Dells, Wisconsin, June 1973.

Miller, J. and Yoder, D.: An ontogenetic language teaching strategy for retarded children. In Lloyd, L. L. and Schiefelbush, R. L. (Eds.): *Language perspectives—Acquisition retardation and intervention.* Baltimore, Maryland: Univ Park, 1974.

Minuchim, P. and Biber, B.: A child development approach to language in the preschool disadvantaged child. *Monogr Soc Res Child Dev, 33*:(8), 1968.

Moores, D. F.: Psycholinguistics and deafness. *Am Ann Deaf, 115*:37-48, 1970.

Pollack, D.: *Educational audiology for the limited hearing infant.* Springfield: Thomas, 1970.

Pollack, D. and Downs, M. P.: A parents guide to hearing aids for young children. *Volta Review 66(10)*:745, 1964.

Reynolds, N. and Risley, T.: The role of social and material reinforcers in increasing talking of a disadvantaged preschool child. *J Appl Behav Analysis. 1*:253-262, 1968.

Russell, K. W., Quigley, S. P., and Power, D. J.: *Linguistics and deaf children.* Washington, D.C.: Alexander Graham Bell Association for the Deaf. 1976.

Schlesinger, I. M.: Production of utterances and language acquisition. In Slobin, D. I. (Ed.): *The ontogenesis of grammar.* New York: Acad Pr, 1971.

Stoller, P. (Ed.): *Black American English.* New York: Dell, 1975.

Stremel, K. and Waryas, C.: A behavioral-psycholinguistic approach to language training. In McReynolds, L. V. (Ed.): Developing systematic procedures for training. Washington, D.C.: *American Speech and Hearing Association Monographs,* No. 18, 96-130, 1974.

Streng, A. H., Kretschmer, R. R., and Kretschmer, L. W.: *Language, learning and deafness.* New York: Grune, 1978.

Wallace, G. and McLoughlin, J. A.: *Learning disabilities, concepts and characteristics.* Columbus, Ohio: Merrill, 1975.

Willbrand, M. L.: Psycholinguistic theory and therapy for initiating two word utterances. *Br J Disord Commun, 12*:37-46, 1977.

Williams, R. and Wolfram, W.: *Social dialects: Differences vs disorders.* Rockville, Maryland: American Speech and Hearing Association, October 1977.

Chapter 6

LANGUAGE INTERVENTION STRATEGIES WITH THE SEVERELY HANDICAPPED

THIS CHAPTER DEALS WITH therapy for children who have severe behavioral limitations, i.e. severely handicapped children. Because the child with severe behavioral limitations needs a full-time program of intervention, the child's caretaker becomes an important part of the team. For this reason, many of the suggestions in this chapter may be useful to the clinician utilizing parents or other aid level people as an extension in the clinical program. Many of the materials and references are of a kind that can be readily interpreted for parents or given to parents as part of their in-service training preparation.

During the latter part of the nineteenth and early part of the twentieth centuries, there was a strong movement toward recognition and protective placement of various severely handicapped persons who were labeled "blind," "deaf," "retarded," etc. This movement was aimed at alleviating the sentence to a life of neglect, mistreatment, and even torture that often fell their lot (Schiefelbusch and Haring, 1976). With the advent of special education and specialized rehabilitation services from the thirties through the fifties, descriptions of methodologies were fairly well label-centered; we found different therapies for persons bearing such labels as cerebral palsy, cleft palate, mental retardation, etc.

During the 1970s, there has been a strong movement away from the use of labels to designate strategies, partly because educational specialists realize that labels do not adequately define specific problems or serve as indicators of methods for intervention; this movement is also a result of public sentiment against "protective" labeling that is morally suspect and ineffective and more often than not compounds the problems of the labeled child (Taylor and Jackson, 1976).

As a consequence, during the past several years there has been a trend away from specialized treatment for categorical labels such as "cerebral palsy" and a broadening of methodologies to overlap categorical boundaries and become more sensitive to the specific needs of each child as an individual. The result has been a movement away from the so-called medical model, which places emphasis upon syndrome labels, and toward the educational model, which emphasizes a problem analysis of each child as the basis for his intervention program.

Specialized Intervention Designs

This emphasis on problem areas as a basis for training has led to a different kind of clustering of children; a grouping that combines children either in terms of problem areas that they have in common or in terms of their response to certain treatment approaches. As a consequence, certain specialized intervention models have emerged and been used with children who respond to these approaches regardless of degree of handicap. These specialized method areas or designs include (1) the sensory-motor drill (or game) emphasis, (2) organismic processing emphasis, (3) the cognitive training emphasis, (4) environmental enrichment emphasis, and (5) behavior modification emphasis. Each of these designs are discussed briefly below. Use of the word *emphasis* suggests that these methods are not completely unique in their content, but rather emphasize somewhat different types of interactions or philosophy.

Sensory-Motor Drill (or Game) Design

This method of training stresses the use of repetition or drill and often utilizes games to make the activities fun and motivating, or to keep the child from "tuning out." The clinician typically gives the child repeated sensory stimuli that call for specific motor responses. This is a simple S-(O)-R-(C) model in which S is the antecedent event or discriminative stimulus; R represents response behaviors; O represents consideration of organismic or individual differences; C stands for consequential events (usually praise or some other type of reward, or perhaps a punishment); italics means this is a most important element; and parentheses indicate that such an element is optional.

The main philosophy behind this method is the traditional belief that "practice makes perfect." An example of this approach is a situation in which the clinician has a set of picture cards portraying familiar objects. The clinician asks the child (O) to name (R) the pictures (S) spontaneously or to imitate the instructor's modeling of the picture names. The objective is to increase the child's labeling repertoire. If the child makes a response, he may be rewarded (C) for his attempt, especially if such attempt is partially or wholly successful.

Organismic Processing Design

This specialized method of approach uses organic processing deficits, such as discrimination or memory deficits, as targets for training. The rationale is that if processing ability is improved, the child will be able to respond to normal learning environments. This model could be described as a S-O-R-(C) method in which modification of the organismic variable facilitates a more normal response. Training activities that are specifically aimed at improving discrimination ability, ability to concentrate, ability to remember, etc., as ways of alleviating organismic processing deficits, fit under this method. Given this approach, the clinician might ask the child (O) to repeat back (R) progressively longer strings of digits or nonsense words (S) and may reward (C) the child for successful responses; the objective of this activity would be to increase the child's auditory memory span (O).

Cognitive Training Design

This method is similar to the one just described and can also be described as an S-O-R-(C) design in which the child's repertoire of knowledge of alternatives that can bring about differing outcomes receives the most important consideration. The O in this design is defined as the knowledge repertoire that the child possesses about how to analyze, problem solve, and make predictions. Most methods that primarily emphasize the development of cognition as the vehicle for more adequate language development would fit under this design.

In this approach, the clinician might present the child (O) with three different valued coins (S) and ask him to tell (R) which is worth more (or will buy more). The objective is for the child to learn to recognize value differences between the coins. His successful responses will likely be followed by some type of praise (C).

Environmental Enrichment Design

This method is somewhat similar to the cognitive training design, except that it is described as S-O-R- (C) with S representing an enriched stimulus climate. (It could include $S_1 + S_2 + S_3$ etc., as part of the stimulus context.) This approach is used mainly with children whose environment is suspected of being impoverished or understimulating, a situation frequently found among the severely handicapped.

In this approach, the clinician might present a contrived experience situation such as "mealtime" or use an actual lunch period as the setting for language training. The stimuli for the language response (s) are multiple, including actual hunger, food, verbal communication, etc. The expected response (R) is for the child to ask for what he wants either spontaneously or as an imitated response, depending upon the response criteria. The child's skill (O) is also considered in setting up the task difficulty; successful responses are likely to be rewarded (C) by presentation of food and/or verbal praise.

Behavior Modification Design

This model includes S- (O)-R-C components like the above models, but has an additional component, K which precedes C. This K represents various contingencies such as schedules of reinforcement, criterion definitions, etc. It is also often expanded to include the O component, which makes allowances for organismic or individual differences but that is an optional component. The components for the full design would therefore be S- (O)-R-K-C.

In this approach, the clinician has as a goal a specific objective and the criteria for relative achievement has been defined. He will present a predetermined stimulus (S), such as a picture or object, and will reward (C) an appropriate response (R) with a predetermined schedule of reinforcement (K); the level of the task difficulty will be determined by the child's base line (R).

There may be other components involved in some models of

training not specified in the above examples, but the various components described probably encompass the major portion of language programs frequently being used.* It is not uncommon for two or more of these methods to be used with the same child.

Individualized Intervention Strategies

Each handicapped person is a unique individual with his own special problems in coping with the demands of his environment. "The *developmental status* of the individual child has been [used as a] basic and cardinal principle: assessment and intervention begin with and end with a consideration of the status and capabilities of the individual child" (Hartup, 1976, pp. 748-749). This point of view has spawned a strong argument against generalized approaches to groups of children who, for one reason or another, have been lumped into a single category. Carl Rogers (1951) was one of the earliest pioneers to recognize the need for individualized planning. He believed that it was the individual, rather than his diagnostic label, that would give valid cues to the necessary direction for remediation. The whole field of special education (including speech and hearing services) has been criticized for its inadequacy in meeting individual needs of its consumers (Valletutti and Grossman, 1976). One of the most frequent criticisms is that diagnostic assessment and evaluation in facilitating the selection of appropriate intervention strategies are inefficient (Ciminero, 1975).

In November 1975, President Ford signed into law PL 94-142, which reflects how critical the issue of individualized planning for intervention is. This law specifically mandates that "the local education agency . . . will establish, or revise, whichever is appropriate, an individualized education program for each handicapped child at the beginning of each school year and will then review and, if appropriate revise, its provisions periodically, but not less than annually" [PL 94-142, Sec. 614 (a) (5)]. No other public law has been as bold nor as specific in prescribing proce-

---

* Fristoe (1975) has provided a brief description of a rather large number of programs available for language training, each of which would fit more or less under one of the above described designs.

dures designed to insure the individual rights of the handicapped child.

A number of preliminary models for developing an individualized instruction program have been presented (see Jackson, 1976 for a review). Generally speaking, individualized educational programming is a dynamic process that might be illustrated by a flow chart like the one in Figure 2. In this chart, the first stage in individualized instruction management would be taking an inventory of the child's present needs. Taking such an inventory requires a relevant and comprehensive assessment procedure. Various forms of assessment, both informal and formal, have been discussed in Chapters 3 and 4.

The severely handicapped probably will require a "team assessment approach," since they will likely have problems in a number of different domains. Assessment on a norm-referenced test will give the clinician a fairly good idea of strengths and weaknesses in terms of a given social setting (i.e. in comparison to a norm group). Results of such assessment, however, will have lit-

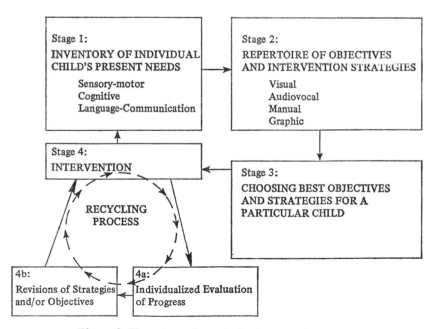

Figure 2. Flow chart through the intervention cycle.

tle to offer in terms of programming objectives for any given child. The criterion-referenced applied behavioral assessment approach probably comes closest to providing a thorough needs-assessment of the competencies that each child needs to try to develop. In addition, the informal procedures discussed in Chapter 4 are essential for adequate individual planning.

The next stage is the process of scanning one's repertoire of knowledge of objectives and possible intervention strategies that might best serve to help the child develop needed competencies. Frequently, clinicians use the so-called normative model as the reference for needed competencies. However, we as yet have only a limited knowledge of what the normative model is in the area of language development. One might use many of the objectives suggested in Chapter 5 as well as in the present chapter for setting up such a model since the severity of handicaps does not always determine what the objectives should be.

A number of curricular programs also are readily available for language training (Fristoe, 1976). *Individualized program planning would preclude using a preprogrammed curriculum per se with any given child.* Such programs, however, usually have a large repertoire of competencies that have been carefully sequenced in terms of difficulty and that may serve as a rich source for selection of objectives for any given child, depending on his needs. Some clients may not benefit from a particular program; it is impossible to determine whether a given subject will benefit from a program or method by use of mean or variance scores from a standardizing group, even though that type of information has been strongly recommended by some professionals (Connell et al., 1977). Mean and variance scores on a representative* group may reveal weak positive effects, even though some members of the group regressed from the treatment; such findings could be misleading and perhaps even dangerous. One can more readily assess the effectiveness of any particular strategy with a given individual by using a method of tracking progress suggested later in this chapter.

The third stage is choosing a beginning set of objectives for

---

* The more representative a sample is the more heterogeneous it becomes and the less representative it is of any single individual (Hersen and Barlow, 1976).

training. An important principle in choosing for severely handicapped is determining ordinal relationships between various objectives in a particular domain and establishing where the child stands in terms of mastery of those ordinal objectives. Often, objectives in a program are rated as to degree of difficulty of mastery or in relative order in which they normally are acquired. This information is very useful for it assists the clinician in zeroing in on the most appropriate level at which to begin treatment.

The fourth stage of the schema for individualized planning is the one called the intervention and evaluation stage in Figure 2. This is possibly the most important part of the intervention model, and probably the most difficult part. The notion of diagnostic teaching as a formal part of the intervention process was earlier suggested by Prouty and Prillaman (1970). Since then it has been implemented in various forms and contexts (Jackson, Lattimore, Hawkins, and Jones, 1976). Intervention evaluation is a closely related concept whose major function is to help the clinician determine which objectives and intervention strategies are working and which are not. In a word, it is a facilitator of decision making relative to the execution of intervention strategies. One major decision to be made in therapy is whether the child is making any progress with particular objectives. Another major decision is the determination of when the child is ready to terminate a particular phase of therapy and move into another level.

The question regarding whether the child is making any progress can be broken down into two parts: *How is the child doing relative to goal mastery? How is the child doing in terms of adjusting to or coping with his environment?*

One can readily answer the first question by setting up criteria for quantitative assessment of goal achievement: a rating scale that gives a judgment of how close the child is to mastery or a frequency of error count in which progress is assessed by computing the percentage of tries that are successful (half-way in goal mastery on a rating scale would be roughly equivalent to 50 percent success on a frequency of success tabulation). Progress on a multiple of goals can be assessed by a minitest called a *probe* in which a small sample of the objectives or goals are assessed for degree of mastery and the results are generalized to the other tasks or goals of a similar nature in the curriculum. The probe is also used to get an idea of the type or degree of movement toward mastery, whether it is slow or fast; a sample of practice sessions over time is selected for assessment of progress toward mastery. The cumulative difference in degree of mastery over time is used as a curve of rate of change or progress; an accelerating curve indicates positive change, a flat line indicates no progress, and a decelerating curve indicates negative change or regression. Steepness of the slope indicates rate of change toward mastery.

These same procedures can be used regardless of whether one is concerned with assessment of progress toward long-range goals or short-range (immediate) goals; but only if proper criterion definitions have been set up relative to quantifying progress.*

The second question regarding progress toward coping with the environment has to do with the ecological relevance of therapy as well as with the progress of the child. The first part of this question is a very difficult one to answer and probably will require some type of inquiry in the form of research. The second part is also difficult to answer but the answer is within reach of the clinician. Ecological "pay off" of therapy can be shown indirectly by looking at the progress the child is making in comparison to other children in the clinician's case load and also by comparing the child with his normal peers from time to time. If he seems to be catching up (or perhaps just staying even), the assumption will be that the therapy has some ecological value. Other indices of ecological value of therapy are improved social adjustment, decreased emotional problems, and improved family relations.

Measures of child-progress help the clinician make decisions as to whether to continue working toward an objective (if the child is making adequate progress but has not yet reached mastery) or to terminate therapy with an objective (if the child has achieved mastery or is not making any progress).

---

* For additional discussion on assessment of progress refer to a later section, "Tracking Progress," of this chapter.

Early Language Objectives for a Nonverbal or Severely Language Delayed Child

Verbal Objectives

Appendix 1 at the end of this chapter contains tables of early language tasks or targets that have been recommended by Ingram and Eisenson (1972) for use with the severely handicapped. The clinician may wish to choose tasks from a repertoire such as this and try various models of intervention (see above for some examples) to see which proves most productive with each individual child. With improved technology, we no longer need place the blame for no progress entirely on the child; it has been demonstrated that some of this blame must rest with the clinician.

Most of the objectives in Appendix 1 are arranged ordinally, i.e. they either proceed from easy to more difficult goals or are arranged in the developmental order in which they typically emerge in children. Such an ordering allows the clinician to determine where to begin; the clinician would do well to probe each of the easier tasks to assess the child's ability to handle each one (percent of successful encounters). The place to begin is probably with those tasks that are somewhere under 90 percent but over 50 percent successful (i.e. transitional tasks); this will insure a greater degree of success, minimal discouragement, and increased motivation. The easier tasks should be mastered first with gradual progression toward the more difficult ones.

The "menu" approach to selecting objectives or behavior targets has more or less emerged from the fair trial philosophy that is based on the premise that each child can learn something; the obligation professionals have to the child is to give him as great an opportunity as possible to demonstrate whether or not he can master specific tasks. Two very important criteria (which overlap to some extent) for making a determination of which tasks to teach first have been suggested by Schiefelbusch, Ruder, and Bricker (1976, p. 275).

1. Train first those language forms and functions that have immediate utility for the child. The word *more*, for example, might have some utility for the child at the one-word stage of development in expressing a request for recurrence of an event (such as "more

cookie" or "more milk"). By focusing on language forms and functions having immediate utility in the child's environment, the [clinician] takes advantage of his readiness for acquiring such a structure and also intrinsically rewards him. This principle may not always be applicable. For instance, it is not always apparent which linguistic structure or class of structure will be useful to a particular individual. Lacking such information, we can turn to the alternate guiding principle.

2. Normal language development data affords at least a reasonable first approximation of what to include in a language training program.

For the severely handicapped child, objectives usually must be broken into very small substeps and, even then, progress is often very slow (Gentry and Haring, 1976). Most curriculum developers suggest that when working with the severely handicapped, tasks should be sequenced through three phases: imitation, comprehension, and spontaneous production (Kent, 1974; Murdock and Hartmann, 1975; Schiefelbusch, Ruder, and Bricker, 1976; Bricker, Ruder, and Vincent, 1976; Mecham, 1977). Detailed instructions are usually provided in the curriculum.

Nonvocal Objectives

For children who do not respond to vocal training, a nonvocal approach to language may prove to be helpful. An example of the type of child likely to be a candidate for this approach is an older nonverbal child who has not responded to oral communication training. Carrier (1976), Bricker (1972), Kent (1972), Kopchick and Lloyd (1976), Topper (1975), Richardson (1975), Wilson (1974), and Kahn (1977) have all reported some success with nonvocal methods of language development with severely and profoundly handicapped children who did not respond to vocal strategies. Whether this is because the speech response system is more complex than manual response systems (Carrier, 1973) or because a higher level of cognition is required for oral communication than for manual communication (Kahn, 1977) can only be speculated. Some studies have reported that development of nonvocal forms of language has had a facilitative effect on the development of vocal language (Hughes, 1972; Creedon, 1974; Shaffer and Goehl, 1974). This combination of nonvocal and vocal systems for language instruction is often referred to as the total communication approach.

Some of the more widely used nonvocal systems for language development include sign languages (Wilbur, 1976), Bliss symbols (Ontario Crippled Children's Center, 1974), Nonspeech Language Initiation Program (Carrier and Peak, 1975; Carrier, 1976), and language boards of various types (Vanderheiden and Grilly, 1976). Most of these systems use logographics (representations of whole words) as the smallest unit. For a more detailed description of some of these systems refer to Appendix 2 at the end of this chapter.

Sign language seems to have some advantage over other nonvocal systems because it appeals to a potentially wider audience and is less cumbersome since it does not require the use of special kits and materials. However, signing is not feasible for many physically handicapped children. Figure 3 suggests some general criteria for use of the various nonvocal systems.

Facilitating Language-Learning Processes

In Chapter 1 we discussed the major processes involved in handling verbal information, such as attention and attentional vigilance, recognition and organization (classification), rehearsal,

Communication Modality	Receptive Skills		Expressive Skills		
	Auditory	Visual	Vocal	Manual	Visual
Sign Language	Poor	Good	Poor	Good	Good
Visual Encoding Board	Poor or Good	Good	Poor	Poor	Good
Visual Scanning Board	Poor or Good	Good	Poor	Poor	Good
Direct Selection Board	Poor or Good	Good	Poor	Good	Good

Figure 3. General criteria for assessing the most feasible nonvocal mode of communication for the nonverbal or unintelligible child. (Excellent descriptions of these various modes of "indicating" in communication are presented by Vanderheiden, 1976.)

and short-term and long-term storage and retrieval. Considerable literature is available describing these processes and their role in handling verbal and other types of information. We will review some literature containing suggestions relative to intervention strategies that might be helpful in improving or alleviating processing deficits that are so likely to be present in the severely CNS impaired child.

Facilitating Attending Behavior

Berry (1969, p. 69) has suggested that we will probably find that in some groups of linguistically handicapped children "interruptions and distortions of auditory perception of the speech continuum are caused mainly by impairment of the set-to-attend mechanism." She also indicated that both span (extensity) and focus (intensity) of attention are important variables in the learning process.

Some of the cues for attentional disturbances that have been described in the literature include distractibility, motor-disinhibition, off-task glancing, and perseveration. If the child demonstrates any of these symptoms, attentional disturbances might be suspected.

Two different approaches may help to remedy attentional disturbances: modification of the environment and modification of the child's attentional adaptation ability. Utilizing both of these approaches would probably be desirable in the intervention program.

Eisenson (1972), Johnson and Myklebust (1967), and others have suggested general procedures that are related to modification of the environment. Multimodal stimulation may load the child's processing mechanisms to overcapacity; limiting sensory stimuli to a single modality* may reduce the input load to better fit the child's capacity. Narrowing down the span (extensity) of the stimuli also helps to reduce the processing load; for example, simple, noncluttered pictures on a plain background are better

---

* Our clinical experience agrees with Eisenson's (1972) suggestion that the visual modality is generally more robust in the severely handicapped than the auditory modality, except in cases of selective visual-modality disturbance. It may therefore be necessary to block out the visual modality in beginning auditory-attention training.

than those with complex or multiple figures on a varied background. Intensification (focus) of stimuli has been suggested as a favorable external variable. Eisenson (1972) suggests intensifying visual stimuli by use of life-size figures and pictures. Earphones and an amplifier can be used to increase the intensity of auditory stimuli.

Familiar materials are better (i.e. will attract attention more readily) than nonfamiliar materials. Objects are better—more concrete—than pictures. Repetition of stimuli may be useful but continual repetition of stimuli presentation may create an adaptation (tuning-out) effect, especially with severe CNS impairment; it is good to avoid prolonged repetition when dealing with children with attentional disturbances.

Two physiological manifestations of attentional disturbance are overactive (exaggerated) orientation response and underactive (weak) orientation response; the former problem may be manifest overtly as hyperactivity (motor disinhibition) and the latter may be manifest by lack of responsiveness in any form. Very little systematic research has been conducted to assess the extent to which attentional skills of the severely handicapped can be changed and the type of attentional training strategies that are effective. More study needs to be done in this area.

Overselective attention is a major problem in severely retarded and autistic children (Wilhelm and Lovaas, 1976); attention is restricted to the most salient part of the stimulus complex and other, less salient, features are ignored. An excellent technique was developed during World War II to increase and broaden selectivity of the momentary attentional store. Tachistoscopic exposures were made of a given number of airplanes appearing simultaneously on one slide; the objective of repeated exposures was to increase the viewer's ability to recognize a progressively larger number of planes in a given length of time. A clinical modification of this technique has been helpful in some cases with moderately handicapped who can recognize and identify pictures. The child is shown a series of cards with varying numbers of pictures (2, 3, 4, etc.) on each card; he is asked to look at the pictures carefully and try to recall them later on. Initially inspection time is usually up to one minute. After presenting a card for a given inspection time, the card is then turned over and the child is asked to name all the pictures he can remember seeing on the card. If the child is nonverbal, he could be shown a series of pictures, only part of which were on the card, and told to indicate whether each was on the original set. Variations of this procedure can be generated by varying the number of pictures on the original cards or varying the inspection time, decreasing it a little at a time.

Encouraging preliminary results have been demonstrated by a study in Utah when another approach (Mecham, 1978) was used with severely handicapped children unable to attend at the Utah State Training School. This approach uses a conditioning paradigm in which the stimulus is presented and the stimulus source is placed immediately in the hand of the child. Frequent pairing of the acoustic and tactile-kinesthetic stimuli seems to strengthen the child's awareness and he begins to react to the acoustic stimulus after initial conditioning has been established. Tactile-kinesthetic stimulation is continued until the visual orientation of looking is established and may then be faded.

Improving Conscious Processing Skills—Rehearsal Srategies

There are a number of phenomena that may be interfering with retention of information in short-term storage. In Chapter 1 we indicated that short-term storage enables one to hold information in consciousness long enough to make a decision regarding what kind of response to make. A number of responses may be made, such as allowing the information to fade from short-term memory without being processed for storage, holding the information in conscious short-term storage indefinitely through "maintenance" or passive-type rehearsal, or processing the information for long-term storage through "elaborative" or active-type rehearsal. Failure in rehearsal strategies appears to be one of the major weaknesses in short-term memory processing for language learning.

Berry (1969, p. 108) has stated that retention problems pervade "every facet of language impairment." She goes on to say that if memory is defective, "language learning and relearning also will be impaired."

The most common types of rehearsal problems seem to be

failure to use any type of rehearsal or repetition, failure to use clustering strategies in rehearsal (i.e. to categorize items being rehearsed according to some commonalities), or failure to use cumulative strategies in rehearsing (i.e. to rehearse previous material two or three times with each new item presented in a series).

Since we assume that attempting to reverse these deficits will have a facilitative effect upon short-term memory processing, it would be well to try to strengthen the child's tendency to use each of these rehearsal strategies as much as possible.

PASSIVE REHEARSAL (IMITATION). We recommend the use of oral imitation as a way of increasing the severely handicapped child's tendency to rehearse, since rehearsal by definition is repetition of verbal material either vocally or subvocally. Establishing an overt imitative repertoire does not insure that the child will generalize this to subvocal rehearsal (which is normally used in more advanced short-term memory processing) but it is reasonable to assume that lack of an imitative repertoire probably insures that the child will not be subvocally rehearsing. On the other hand, repetition training has been found to improve children's learning performance (Flavell, 1970).

In the piagetian sense, the form of imitation most easily elicited is where the patterns that the model presents for the child to imitate are patterns that the child has spontaneously and frequently produced himself previously. In the normal infant, this type of imitation occurs early in the sensory-motor stage (age four to eight months). The type of patterns to be modeled for the child to imitate at this stage should be dictated by close observation of spontaneous vocal patterns frequently being emitted by the child. This will necessitate observing the child during some fairly representative samples of his social contacts.

Later (eight to twelve months) the child will be able to imitate novel constructions. Early imitations of this type commonly encouraged are voluntary opening and closing of the mouth (Morehead and Morehead, 1974) and producing words having highly visible sound elements such as *papa* and *mama*. Single words may be more readily elicited at first,* followed by simple word cou-

---

* Vocal imitation may need to be preceded by establishment of a nonvocal motor or gesture repertoire (for procedures see Baer, Peterson, and Sherman, 1967).

plets. According to Berry (1969, p. 149) a child "does not readily attend to single phonemes because such attention interferes with comprehension." It is therefore better to work with holistic patterns such as words or short phrases.

Some have argued that imitation is not necessarily involved in the language acquisition of normal children (McNeill, 1970; Menyuk, 1963). However, if imitation is found useful as a special language intervention procedure for establishing a verbal repertoire in severely handicapped, whether or not it is a necessary condition in normal language acquisition becomes somewhat irrelevant (Bricker and Bricker, 1974).

REHEARSAL AS AN ORGANIZATION PROCESS (CLUSTERING). Undergirding the development of concepts and meaning is the process of clustering or categorizing. Words and phrases are labels that come to represent these categories. The taxonomic process is the main means for organizing our world conceptually and for deriving, from dynamic categorical relationships, the operations that become known as abstract thinking. "A person who defines an apple tree as a tree and a goat as an animal disregards the attribute peculiar to an apple tree or goat and isolates some essential quality of each that pertains to a generic category" (Luria, 1976, p. 84).

Memory span experiments have shown that the capacity of the short-term memory store is limited and that seven units of information (plus or minus two) seems to be the average storage capacity of adults (Miller, 1956; Johnson, 1970; Loftus and Loftus, 1976); they have further shown that if information units having similar characteristics are clustered into one unit, this unit can be stored as a single item and upon retrieval can again be broken down into its component units (Johnson, 1970). Thus, the process of chunking or clustering for short-term storage makes it possible for us to hold in short-term memory store seven or so clusters each containing up to seven separate items of information. We know that adults can repeat back sentences with more than seven to nine words. The assumption is that clusters of words are stored in either syntactic or sentence units.

The process of clustering for short-term memory is less efficient if the clusters are very similar in character; it is maximally efficient if the clusters are highly dissimilar. For example, one can retain two clusters more readily if one contains letters and the other one contains numbers than if both contained the same type of items such as letters. Proactive interference in short-term retention occurs when an item to be stored is preceded by the item similar in characteristics; it is released (or reduced) when the item to be stored is preceded by a taxonomically dissimilar item in the stimulus chain (Wickens, 1972; Cody and Borkowski, 1977).

Since chunking or clustering is such a powerful device in assimilating, storing, relating, and retrieving information for language learning, developing improved clustering or grouping skills is an important remedial objective for severely language handicapped who are having trouble in this area. (Evaluation of the child's ability to chunk and categorize was discussed in Chapter 3.) Some common subobjectives that relate very closely to and are probably involved in clustering and chunking are figure-ground differentiation, stimulus recognition and constancy, and abstracting (i.e. relating various clusters into a single higher order category). We will give some general suggestions relative to remedial planning for each of these and suggest resources for the detailed procedures that have been presented.

Auditory figure-ground differentiation is the process of screening out the more salient (or important) elements of a stimulus complex and ignoring (or giving secondary attention to) other remaining stimuli. One of the first evidences of figure-ground differentiation manifested by an infant is the appearance of hand watching behavior; the infant may fixate on his hands or follow them with his eyes as they move out of sight. If the infant reaches for an object with the intent of grasping it, this suggests he is developing figure-ground differentiation—the figure (the hand) is the most salient stimulus set and its surroundings become unimportant or ignored. Auditorily, an infant manifests selective attention to a specific sound within a background of random auditory stimuli. An important clue to this differentiation can be seen in localized behaviors of the child, such as looking in the direction of the sound source or locating in a multiple choice situation the source of a particular sound among a number of possible sources (e.g. upon hearing a drum, the child sees a drum, xylophone, and whistle and focuses on the drum since it was the source of the sound he heard). Another indication of acoustic figure-ground discrimination is when the child indicates he differentiates angry or pleasant speech from his caretaker and reacts by either crying or smiling, whichever is appropriate. A more advanced stage of auditory figure-ground recognition is manifested by the child if he listens to noise makers on a tape or record with background noise and points to pictures of the noise being made (e.g. dog bark, telephone ring, auto horn, etc.). The auditory testing and training record by Utley (1950) is an excellent example of training procedures for facilitating auditory figure-ground differentiation.

Early experiences of children involve interactions with things and actions and variability of things and actions. Common noun (things) categories that develop in severely limited children as a result of early experiences are *bed, blanket, brother, candy, chair, clean, coat, comb, cookie, cup, daddy, dirty, dog, drink, eat, fork, glass, home, kitty, knife, milk, mama, pants, pillow, plate, shirt, shoe, soap, sack, spoon, table, teeth, toilet, towel, TV, water.* Vygodsky (1962) has said that "The sensory material and the world are both inseparable parts of concept formation" (p. 52). As a rule, the label is paired frequently with the experience and usually becomes part of the concept of the experience (Mecham, 1969). A programmed book on auditory perceptual training by Reagan (1973) includes a section on figure-ground differentiation training.

Stimulus recognition and object permanence is a stage of perceptual development that immediately follows figure-ground differentiation. One of the earliest indicators that a child recognizes an object and its meaning is proper use-manipulation, e.g. taps a drum, shakes a bell, clangs the cymbols, puts bottle in mouth. Once an object has acquired a state of permanence, the child recognizes it in various contexts and in various sizes, colors, and (to some extent) shapes. At this time he also is aware of the disappearance of a hidden object and looks searchingly for it.

Stages of recognition and object permanence can be encouraged by teaching the child to interact properly with objects through appropriate manipulation. It is helpful in the language training situation, if labeling accompanies the child's actual recognition of objects and situations. Recognition of meaningful interaction concepts is often easier for the child if he recognizes the various subjects or objects related to the concepts. Leonard (1975) demonstrated this by having an assistant model responses to simple commands and found that retarded children learned concepts and concept labels much more readily if they were illustrated or demonstrated in situational contexts. Words and phrases describing general semantic relations such as *agent, dative, instrument, and object* were especially more readily learned as a part of a situational context.

Bricker and Bricker (1970, 1974, 1976), Bricker, Dennison, Watson, and Smith (1973), Miller and Yoder (1974), and Maharaj (1975) are among those who stress development of object recognition and permanence as an early intervention strategy for severely language delayed children.

Abstratcting is the process of including various concepts under a single higher level classification—it is a process of leaving out details. In the process of abstracting, concepts such as *bed, blanket,* and *pillow,* for example, are eventually associated together under a general class of "sleeping" or "night-night." *Clean, comb, dirty, soap, teeth, toilet, towel,* and *water* may be associated under the general class of "cleanliness" or "grooming"; *candy, cookie, cup, drink, fork, glass, knife, mouth, plate, spoon,* and *table,* may all become related under the general concept of "eating" or "feeding." They are related to such categories only after repeated experiences have been encountered by the child relating the items in a certain way. This process of viewing different items in terms of the same or similar function is referred to by Piaget as assimilation (1973, p. 70). Variability of actions and objects or agents are usually assimilated into general concepts of how things and actions differ, e.g., see the following (Mecham, 1969): (1) The general concept of "time" includes more elementary concepts such as already, early, late, recent, soon, today, always, since, etc. (2) The general concept of "color" includes various specific color concepts with which we are all familiar, labeled with various color words. (3) The general concept of "manner" includes such specific concepts as active, funny, lazy, serious, mean, strong, etc. (4) The general concept of "distance" includes specific concepts such as further, near, here, far, long, close, etc. (5) The "number" class includes such specific concepts as various specific numbers, both, many, none, etc. (6) the general class labeled "shape" includes all of the possible shapes encountered in the early experiences of the child such as round, square, etc. (7) The classification of "amount" could encompass such concepts as equal, many, all, full, half, much, some, etc. Other classifications include "size," "direction," "temperature," and "quality."

The clinician may notice that the above classifications or abstractions are closely tied to various modalities such as auditory, visual, or tactile-kinesthetic. More abstract categories that are not modality dependent include such concepts as concern, responsibility, acceptance, etc.

A rule of thumb for estimating level of abstraction is to ask how much agreement occurs between two listeners in respect to specific modal-imagery when they hear the label for the concept. Two persons who hear the term *apple pie* will have a very similar modal-imagery of vision, smell, and taste. If they hear the term *animal,* however, they will differ extensively as to the imagery that occurs; one will say she saw a "little white dog," while the other may say she saw a "gray kitty," etc. The higher the level of abstraction, the greater the variety of possible specific or detailed descriptions.

It is important to consider the above rule of thumb in the sense that more concrete classifications are less variable, more imagery bound, and thus are more easily grasped and retained by the severely handicapped child. It is therefore better to work with the various concepts of variability that are part of the child's modal-image world first and then move into higher levels of abstraction wherever possible. Basic constructions (see Chapter 1) in language tend to be easier for the child to learn in the early language experience than more complex and variable transformations. It is probably for this reason that during the early phases many language training programs for the severely handicapped deal predominantly with base structure (Kent, 1972; Mecham, 1977).

The clustering strategy in learning enables the child to band new meanings into some categorical system or to tie together various already learned meanings into a new category. Clustering is the most effective rehearsal strategy for these children since it helps the meaning or semantic aspect of language to be learned and used. A different kind of learning is required for committing to long-term memory the formal or structural aspects of perceptions. This requires some type of rote memorization and depends upon the type of rehearsal discussed in the next section.

CUMULATIVE REHEARSAL SKILLS. Cumulative rehearsal is a different strategy than the clustering-type rehearsal described above. In clustering rehearsal, the child groups items together in terms of some common property or function. In cumulative rehearsal, the child rehearses items in sequence over and over with the purpose in mind of committing them to the type of storage that will allow them to be retrieved in their exact same form. Piaget refers to this type of learning as accommodation. Whereas imitation is a form of passive accommodation (see above), cumulative rehearsal is an active or elaborative type of accommodation and appears to be the most powerful means of learning and remembering detailed structure characteristics and arbitrary rules such as we find in language syntax. Reichart, Cody, and Borkowski (1975) found that cumulative rehearsal was much more efficient for retarded persons in committing serial lists to memory than the clustering-type rehearsal. In its most effective form, the clinician has the child repeat recently learned material two or three times with each new item to be learned; thus the strength of retention builds up cumulatively over a number of rehearsal sessions.

Cumulative rehearsal strategies are relatively common in language training programs where familiar objects or pictures are presented for the child to name or describe prior to introducing a new object or picture; when the new object or picture becomes familiar, it then becomes part of the series for cumulative rehearsal in future therapy sessions.

Reichart, Cody, and Borkowski (1975) listed the various rehearsal strategies in order of relative effectiveness in committing verbal materials to both short-term and long-term memory as follows: (1) Passive clustering (in which items are clustered according to some commonality but the child is not informed of their commonality) was not effective. (2) Active clustering (in which the subject was asked to rehearse ways in which items of a cluster are similar) was effective. (3) Cumulative clustering (in which both cumulative and clustering rehearsal strategies were encouraged) was an effective method. (4) Cumulative rehearsal (in which no category event was involved) was most effective in rote recall.

Although the above discussion of facilitation of language-learning processes is not exhaustive, it may serve to stimulate clinicians to investigate these areas and incorporate processing-training in the therapy program for those children who are suspected of having processing problems.

Tracking Progress

Reports of success in using a particular language intervention strategy or preprepared program may be important in the initial selection of programs for the clinician's general resource bank (Connell, Spradlin, and McReynolds, 1977); however, reports of success with others (no matter how impressive) do not insure that the strategy or program you have chosen will be successful with the child you are working with. Each goal has to be monitored closely and objectively by the clinician to determine the extent of progress being made at the moment and/or over a specified period of time. The intervention procedures or programs you are using are valuable to you only if progress is being made by you toward a particular objective for a particular child at a particular time. In tracking clinical progress, you must keep data. "Data collection is justifiable when it leads to the modification of instruction programming that facilitates the individual's progress. However, data which are collected but not used to benefit the child are a costly waste of resources" (Gentry and Haring, 1976, p. 210).

Perhaps even more important than selecting standardized intervention strategies or programs is using standardized measurement procedures; this will insure that valid and reliable judgments are secured concerning the influence of any therapeutic procedure.

The purpose of the following discussion is to present some standard measurement guidelines for the clinician assessing the progress being made by the child.

Types of Measures

Various types of evaluation can be used as part of the planning and implementation of clinical intervention (Gronlund, 1977). One important kind used for evaluating a child's readiness for entry into a particular type and sequence of instruction is called placement evaluation; this is normally used prior to the child's entry into the program. A second type of evaluation that enables the clinician to determine approximately what kind of training the child needs or what kind of objectives need to be set up is called diagnostic evaluation; this centers around the determination of types of behavioral problems or disorders that are interfering with the child's adjustment. A third type of evaluation allowing the clinician to monitor progress of a child during the intervention process is called formative evaluation. A criterion-referenced test and/or informal language sampling procedures (see Chapter 4) are more appropriate and sensitive than any kind of norm-referenced test since progress is assessed by comparing a child's behavior against the criterion set up for each target objective. A fourth type of evaluation allows one to assess progress by the child over a substantial time span and over a broad spectrum of performance domains, this is called summative evaluation (it can involve both norm-referenced and criterion-referenced tests).

Both formative and summative types of evaluation are helpful in measuring the progress a child is presently making (formative) or has already made in the past (summative). Each of these types of evaluation will be mentioned only briefly here (for a more detailed discussion see Gentry and Haring, 1976).

Formative assessment helps the clinician know whether the child "is making progress, whether or not his rate of progress is adequate, or whether he has mastered one learning task and is ready to advance to another" (Gentry and Haring, 1976, p. 210). Precise and sensitive measurement of progress can be invaluable in assessing the relative efficiency of various methods of instruction being used (Hersen and Barlow, 1976).

In order for progress data to be meaningful, they must be sensitive and comparable to some existing standard concerning ultimate outcome (such a standard is called the criterion for mastery of the target behavior in question). Some basic requirements for utilizing formative-type assessment have been suggested. Gentry and Haring (1976) suggested that (1) the measurement should be taken directly on the task or objective being taught; (2) the measurement should provide information about the intended or critical outcome; (3) the measurement needs to be sensitive enough to reflect change (the larger the number of units in a scale, generally the more sensitive it is to change); (4) measures should be taken frequently (usually a short probe at each therapy session); (5) the measurement should be reliable; (6) the measurement should be practical, e.g. it should not consume an undue amount of intervention time; and (7) the measurement should be efficient and economical (i.e. a large amount of information should be received in return for a small amount of effort and expense). One can select any type of measurement that meets these criteria; or, if such measures are not available, the clinician may wish to develop her own.

Summative assessment measures the progress the child has made over a wide spectrum of performances and/or over an extended period of time. Summative tests can be either norm-referenced (comparing the child's standing with that of his normal peers both before and after training) or criterion-referenced (describing the tasks the child *can* and/or *cannot* perform). Norm-referenced tests by design usually cover a broad number of objective domains and/or age levels and contain a rather small number of objectives under each domain or age level; criterion-referenced tests by design usually cover a narrow range of domains and samples and contain a large number of objectives under each domain. For this reason, the criterion-referenced test is usually much more sensitive to small units of change.

Recording Observations

One of the least standardized and yet most crucial parts of intervention for the speech pathologist is his method of recording observations. Traditional anecdotal notes, written occasionally and specifying simple '"progress" or "no progress," are not presently considered appropriate or credible methods of recording progress (this is especially important wherever progress is extremely slow). Recording that the child made three correct responses out of twenty trials in the beginning and eighteen correct responses out of twenty trials at the end of a training period, however, would probably be appropriate and credible, assuming that conditions for beginning and final observations were comparable (i.e. same constraints, opportunities, and time factors). It goes without saying that a clinician could not remember comparative occurrences or even percentages of relative success observed on a number of occasions during treatment; such occurrences or percentages should be recorded along with some qualitative description of the contexts and nature of the testing or probe procedures. Numerous behavior observation recording systems have been suggested (Mowrer, 1971; Diedrich, 1973; Gelfand and Hartmann, 1975; Gentry and Haring, 1976; White and Liberty, 1976; Kent and Foster, 1977; etc.).

The type of system one uses will depend upon the types of observation (i.e. frequency, latency, duration, trials to criterion, etc.) being made and one's own preference as to whether one wishes to tabulate, chart, or use observer ratings (the latter choice is probably least desirable since it is the most expensive, least objective, and least sensitive type of measure of behavior fluctuations).

Importance of Baseline Data

In order to establish that the child is making more progress with the advent of intervention than he would without, it is important to establish a baseline, which consists of a series of observations (repeated measures) of the target behavior during a nonintervention (usually preintervention) period—often referred to as phase A of the intervention program. The purpose of the baseline is to serve as a measure of the behavior change that may be expected by chance. Such expectation can then be compared to a series of measures during intervention—phase B of the program—and discrepancies between the phase A curve (baseline) and phase B curve (progress line) can indicate whether changes under phase B are greater than one would expect by chance. This design for assessing change is a very powerful tool for determining effectiveness of therapy; it can also be used as a method for assessing relative efficacy of various methods (or variations) of therapy with any given individual.

The use of multiple baselines greatly increases the efficiency of assessing effects of therapy. In this approach, one establishes a baseline over a number of observations for several possible target behaviors (such as verb inflections, prepositions, and articulation) against which changes can be evaluated. It is then possible to intervene with one of those target behaviors and establish whether there is a difference in the phase A and phase B curves for that behavior but not for the others. If one finds a change in only the target behavior, this is even more convincing evidence that it is therapy that is effecting the change (Hersen and Barlow, 1976). Moreover, if a change in the other targets corresponds precisely in time with the advent of introduction of intervention, one can confidently assume it is the intervention rather than the "Hawthorne" effect that is responsible for the change.

Pseudoprogress Precautions

Liberty and White (1976) have outlined some pseudoprogress precautions to be considered during the formative assessment process; the clinician should be cognizant of them and take them into consideration when making an assessment.

THE CONSTRAINT VARIABLE. Changes in constraints or freedom to respond may make it look like the child is improving. For example, if the child is constrained by an emotional upset on the day of the pretest, it may look like he has improved because he communicates better on the posttest and the change may be attributed to intervention when in fact it was due to chance variability of the child.

THE OPPORTUNITY VARIABLE. If the child asks two locative questions (for example, "Where is the ball?") on one day and ten the second day, it will look like he has improved in use of locative expressions; this improvement may be attributed to intervention, especially if intervention has been directed toward use of locatives. The improvement, however, may not be improvement at all, but may merely be the result of difference in opportunity or incentive to use locatives.

THE TIME VARIABLE. Language samples taken on the same child on two different occasions may appear to be different in terms of total number of utterances recorded, i.e. the presample may have only 20 utterances while the postsample may contain 100 utterances. It might appear that the child is much more fluent on the posttest. However, unless the time element is equal for each sample, this conclusion could be erroneous. In order to make a judgment of fluency improvement, one must insure that the time period covered on the presample and postsample are equal.

Decision to Discontinue or Change a Target Objective or Training Strategy

When should one give up (discontinue) a target objective due to lack of progress? Since progress is often very slow and pinpointed, one should, first of all, make sure that the objective has been broken down into very small steps in order to maximize the child's likelihood of success, motivation, and gradual movement toward the objective-criterion. If rate of progress is much slower than one feels is acceptable, the target objective can be broken down into finer steps, changed to another objective within the same domain (e.g. vocabulary acquisition), or discontinued and replaced with an objective in a different domain (e.g. change from vocabulary building to phrase comprehension or production).

In the event no objectives are achieved in a particular modality over a rather substantial trial period (e.g. no audiovocal behaviors within a six to twelve month training period), one may make a decision to attempt a different modality (for example, sign language or Bliss symbolics).

In some instances, lack of progress in any modality may cue the clinician to look at domains other than communication, such as prelanguage cognitive training, as a needed area of acquisition prerequisite to communicative development. In this case, it may well be that the team of professionals working with the child will deem cognitive training more important than overt communication at the moment and recommend discontinuing overt communication training. In such cases, where a decision must be made as to whether to continue or discontinue a specialized area of training (such as self-help, communication, or academics), it should be the right of the child or his surrogate to require a "team" decision involving a panel of advocates. Even if a team decision is not *required* for such an important matter, the clinician probably will still feel more comfortable and less vulnerable to litigation if a team is involved in every case.

Working with Ancillary Behaviors

A child with severe behavioral limitations cannot easily generalize behaviors being taught in one domain and coordinate them with behaviors being taught in another domain, especially if these domains are being taught by different persons. Since treatment of the severely limited child should not be fragmented by different services being offered by different people, it behooves the clinician to be aware of and even be able to do supportive teaching in areas that are typically the province of other professions—such as, the psychologist (behavior modification), the physical therapist (locomotion and gross motor skills), the teacher (academic and/or cognitive skills), and the parent (cleanliness and grooming). The teacher and the parent are often the only members of the team who are assigned to carry out "hands on" training in all domains with the child at school and at home. The clinician needs to not only be aware of what activities the teacher and parent may be involved in and how these can be coordinated with language training activities, but should also be in a position to assist the teacher and parent in language training and other ancillary behaviors when necessary. In some locations, especially in rural areas or areas that cannot afford intensive resources, the teacher, parent, and speech pathologist may be the only members of the team responsible for planning and implementing an individualized program for severely limited children. The speech pathologist frequently is chosen over other specialized resources because severe behavioral limitation is a major social problem for the child and family, and language and communication are the behaviors that are most likely to help to counteract the social breach resulting from the severe handicap.

The speech pathologist working with severely handicapped must orient himself toward treating the whole child, which may involve trying to help the child overcome such things as temper tantrums, head banging, toilet accidents, poor self-feeding, or self-dressing skills; this is done in addition, or adjunctively, to language and communication training (Spradlin and Spradlin, 1976).

Moreover, as stated frequently in this chapter, the clinician may be mainly serving in the capacity of planner-advisor-supervisor to parents and/or other direct care personnel. The "traditional model of removal for an hour of therapy per week will not result in success with the target population of severely impaired children. Rather than use this model, we believe that those individuals with the child should be trained to deliver the necessary special services" (Bricker, 1976). The following sections present suggestions for training in areas of social behaviors closely allied to language and communication behavior.

Elimination of Interfering Behaviors

There are a number of resources available regarding procedures for reducing stereotyped behaviors (Spradlin, Girardeau, and Corte, 1966; Hollis, 1967; Lovaas and Simmons, 1969; Foxx and Azarin, 1973). The procedure suggested by Foxx and Azarin involving overcorrection has been successfully used by a number of people. This procedure utilizes overcorrection as both an aversive consequence of stereotyped behavior and as an incompatible response. An example of the procedure for chronic head-rolling behavior is given. The overcorrection consisted of "functional movement training for five minutes each time the child rolled her head. Initially the [clinician] used [his] hands to restrain the child's head. The [clinician] then told the subject to move her head in one of three positions. For example, 'turn head up.' If the child did not move her head in the desired direction immediately, the clinician manually guided her head. After a time the child would move her head in response to verbal direction. Then the child was required to hold her head still for 15 seconds and a new command was given" (p. 247).

Teaching Self-Help Skills

Self-help training involves teaching such skills as toileting, washing, dressing, grooming, and feeding in a more acceptable manner. The lack of such skills will often prevent social and educational interactions. Brief descriptions of training procedures and some references to more extended study will be presented below for each of these areas. Clinicians should capitalize on opportunities to verbally model appropriate language to describe each activity; verbalization should be kept simple and geared to child's language stage.

TRAINING IN TOILETING. One of the first steps is to determine percentage of appropriate versus inappropriate eliminations in order to get a base level. Procedures for working with toilet training skills have been suggested by Azarin et al. (1971) and Mahoney et al. (1971), and they have been summarized by Spradlin and Spradlin (1976). Both Azarin and Mahoney have developed devices for immediate detection of wetting accidents. The devices developed by Azarin et al. (1971) are available commercially for about $40.00 each.* They can also be constructed for not more than $10.00. The first device has two metal snaps that are attached to the child's cotton panties. The snaps are connected by two small wires to a circuit box mounted on a small belt around the child's waist. When wetness provides an electric circuit between the two metal snaps, a high frequency tone is emitted from the circuit box; the tone can be heard by both the trainer and the child (trainee). A device operating on this same principle has been developed and can be attached to the potty-chair. When moisture is produced, the high frequency noise can be heard immediately.

A prescriptive program for toilet training, which can be used by parents or other supportive personnel, is included as part of the CAMS program (Casto, 1977).

CLEANLINESS AND GROOMING. Cleanliness is also a trait that has a strong influence upon social acceptability of the child. According to Spradlin and Spradlin (1976) cleanliness training should

---

* The device developed by Azarin et al. can be obtained from Lehigh Valley Electronics, Inc., Box 125, Fogelsville, Pennsylvania 18051.

be carried out wherever it is customary for a child to wash, e.g. after playing outside, after toileting, and prior to snacks or lunch. If taught under these contexts, they become stronger discriminative stimuli for cuing washing at appropriate times. Frequent inspection at appropriate times will enable the clinician or parent to determine the extent to which the child is practicing the washing habit. If allowing the child to participate in lunch or snack time is contingent upon prior washing, the tendency for the child to wash at these times will be greatly increased. If the child is not given the snack privilege when he fails to wash, he will be more prone to wash next time to avoid missing the snack.

Spradlin and Spradlin (1976) have reminded us that proper use of the handkerchief and control of drooling are excellent targets for training in children who are lacking in these two areas. "Once again, a child should not be allowed to engage in reinforcing activities . . . if he is drooling or has failed to use his handkerchief properly. Moreover, in some cases it will be necessary to teach the child step-by-step how to wipe his nose, his chin, and other parts of his body" (p. 251). Cleaning fingernails and teeth and grooming the hair may also become important targets for cleanliness training (Casto, 1977).

OTHER SELF-HELP SKILLS. Breland (1965), Baker et al. (1973, 1976), and Casto (1977) have all developed excellent programs that can serve as guides to clinicians and parents in the area of dressing skills for the severely handicapped. These curricula cannot be presented to all children in the same way, but they can serve as a relatively broad band memo of target behavior that could easily be adapted to individual children.

Spradlin and Spradlin (1976) have indicated that "Teaching a child self-dressing skills appears simple until attempted—then it immediately becomes complex" (p. 252). One problem is "reinforcing the child precisely when he [is] engaged in the right movement." Another problem can stem from slight differences in procedures between different trainers. With one child, for example, two trainers used exactly the same sequence of steps in training him self-dressing skills; one trainer, however, started the sequence with the right hand of the child, while the other one started it with his left hand. "When the trainers worked out

these [differences], training went [much more] smoothly"
(p. 252).

A number of reports have suggested procedures for teaching
self-feeding skills with the severely handicapped. Rather detailed
suggestions have been given by Spradlin (1964), Whitney and
Barnard (1966), Henrickson and Doughty (1967), Bartin, Guess,
Garcia and Baer (1970), O'Brien, Bugle, and Azrin (1972),
Baker et al. (1973, 1976) and Casto (1977); and these have provided target objectives in their prescriptive programs especially
designed for parents.

O'Brien and Azrin suggested three types of strategies to be
used depending on the ability of the child to respond: (1) instructions only, (2) instructions with modeling to be imitated,
and (3) instructions plus manually guiding the movements the
child goes through for self-feeding. This latter method is probably imperative in the beginning training with the profoundly
handicapped and may also be necessary with less handicapped
when training concerns the proper use of utensils for eating.

Training in Simple Comprehension and Imitating

Social behavior training involves very importantly the development of ability to comprehend simple greetings and instructions.
Learning to respond to greetings or to carry out simple instructions may require training in imitative behavior. "Imitation is
not considered a great skill for children who imitate. However,
we need only look at a child who doesn't imitate to see its importance" (Spradlin and Spradlin, 1976, p. 254).

The beginning training in comprehending communication is
accompanied by imitative training. When one "starts from
scratch" in comprehension training, it is usually necessary to teach
not only comprehension of simple instructions, but also ways in
which the child can manifest his understanding of those instructions, vis-à-vis by actually carrying them out. For example, the
clinician says, "Where is the ball?" and simultaneously points to
the ball. If the child makes an approximation of imitating the
pointing gesture when he hears "where is the ball," he is reinforced and the tendency for such imitation will be strengthened.
Baer, Peterson, and Sherman (1967) described a procedure for

establishing imitative behavior in the severely retarded children. This procedure has been used many times to establish imitative behavior among retarded and autistic children (Spradlin and Spradlin, 1976, p. 254).

Once imitation of the clinician has been established, carry-over of imitation can be facilitated by having the child learn to imitate the parent and also other children in the school. Such carry-over or generalization will be extremely helpful for much of the social learning that can go on in the classroom, such as sitting on appropriate chairs, engaging in coloring and drawing, taking off coats and hanging them up, or putting on coats in preparation for going outside. Imitation of simple command responses needs to be generalized also to the parent and teacher. Garcia (1974) demonstrated that learning of simple comprehension and communicative behaviors do not generalize into home and classroom situations but have to be taught in those contexts; it is therefore important for the parent and the teacher to carry out in the home and the classroom the same instructional comprehension training and corresponding imitation of proper responses as are being taught by the clinician.

One study demonstrated the utility of having a third person, perhaps the parent, do the modeling of the response to be imitated (Leonard, 1975). The clinician would say "sit down" and the third person would sit and be visibly reinforced while the child is watching. Leonard found that such procedure greatly facilitated getting the child to imitate in order to receive the same rewarding consequences—the consequences might be verbal praise or food reinforcement, etc.

Simple instructions or commands should be accompanied by as many contextual clues as possible, for example, when the clinician says "sit down" he gestures with his hand and glances away from the child toward the chair. Such accompanying clues serve to enrich the stimuli for cuing a proper response and can become substitutes for previously utilized imitative responses.

Perceptual-Motor Training

"Many children with severe behavioral limitations will have trouble crawling, walking or running. Few of these children will exhibit the gross perceptual motor skills needed to enjoy games. Most will not be able to catch or throw a ball with accuracy. Many will also have problems with finer perceptual motor tasks such as putting pegs in holes, working puzzles, and putting taps on bolts" (Spradlin and Spradlin, 1976, p. 225).

A number of resources are available for the clinician to use in becoming more familiar with procedures and objectives for perceptual-motor training. These include writings of such people as Cheney and Kephart (1968), Cratty (1968, 1972), Reger (1970), Finnie (1970), Jones (1974, 1978), Baker et al (1976), Casto (1977), and Popovich (1977).

Interdisciplinary Intervention

Single disciplines have a limited capacity to deal with the myriad problems of the severely and profoundly handicapped. Theoretically, a consortium of intervention specialists could act together and more adequately generate an intervention program that would transcend the scope of any single specialty. There are presently fairly strong pressures for the development and maintenance of the so-called team approach to dealing with the severely and profoundly handicapped. The team approach is favored, for example, by the Accreditation Council for Facilities for the Mentally Retarded *Standards for Residential Facilities for the Mentally Retarded.* Many residential facilities have adopted what is referred to as the unit system, which is another term for the team concept.

In the team model, the speech pathologist, audiologist, physical therapist, occupational therapist, social worker, psychologist, and teacher (or direct care person) act together in the planning and implementation of an intervention program for each individual child. What frequently happens, however, is that each team member examines the child separately, makes a diagnosis, and suggests target intervention objectives that relate specifically to his own discipline. The group then get together for "staffing" of the various problems and objective areas and come up with a multifaceted program for the child. This has been referred to by Gallagher et al. (1976) as a multidiscipline model and does not do much to transcend the scope of any one single discipline.

The strong forces that tend to perpetuate the multidisciplinary model and make the truly interdisciplinary model difficult are things like "territoriality, professional status, identity, and recognition and rewards" (Hartup, 1976, p. 747). The multidisciplinary influence is seen even in preprepared programs such as the "Read Project" or the "CAMS programs"; we find separate booklets written by specific disciplinarians on such things as speech and language training, feeding training, perceptual-motor training, etc. The program, however, that perhaps comes closest to utilizing an interdisciplinary rather than a multidisciplinary approach is the one used in the Portage Project (Shearer and Shearer, 1976) developed to help meet needs for preschool training in a rural area that cannot afford the luxury of a multidisciplinary team. This set of guidelines was developed to be used by parents in the home to teach preschool children under the supervision of a "home teacher." Although it is partially disciplinarian in nature, it is broken down into the areas of cognition, self-help, motor, socialization, and language; it is based on normal developmental growth patterns, is heavily behaviorally oriented, and is geared mainly for parents who are not oriented to any particular discipline.

The factor in the educational setting that cannot be fragmented along the lines of professional disciplines is the child. One way to transcend the influence of the single disciplines running parallel to each other, each getting his own share of the child, is to train interventionists equally as thoroughly in all disciplines relating to child behavior. Until the day comes when this occurs, and it will probably be a long time in coming, various members of the team should try to view the child's problems as the central elements that determine what objectives and intervention strategies should be undertaken.

"Truly interdisciplinary [intervention] would be conducted only when independent variables were identified within other disciplines. For example, if one manipulates a psychological variable such as task instructions and measured such variables as GSR, EKG, or some other physiological measure, then one would be about the business of biopsychology. It is such studies that create useful linkages between usually discrete bodies of knowledge and that allow a fuller examination of that trite but relevant term 'the whole child' " (Gallagher et al., 1976, p. 181).

Use of Supportive Personnel and Parents

With the development of behavior modification procedures and technology in programming, it is now possible to use parents and other "aide" level persons as an extension of the clinical person. Using programmed procedures allows the clinician to provide daily contact with clients through the use of supportive personnel—contacts as frequently and for as long a time-period as each client warrants. There are a number of programs available for use by parents and other aides from which the clinician can draw. If objectives can be selected from such programs, there is the added advantage that suggested procedures for supportive personnel to follow have already been worked out, usually by persons who have been trained in behavior modification and in programming precise procedures to be followed.* Operant programs for language intervention with retarded children that can be used by parents and other aides under supervision of the clinician have been listed and briefly described by Fristoe (1975, 1976).†

There are also current programs dealing with all areas of training that may be used by parents and aides under the supervision of a professional staff. These include CAMS programs (Casto, 1977), *Steps to Independence Series* (Baker et al., 1976), and *Prescriptive Behavioral Checklist* (Popovich, 1977).

Supportive Personnel

Today, supportive personnel are found in almost every setting where severely handicapped are being educated—residential schools for the deaf or mentally retarded, speech and hearing clinics, and public school classrooms. Aides and attendants in institutions have been functioning in educative roles for years; their roles in schools and clinics have been a fairly recent de-

---

* Some trainers have found more successful parent follow-through when expectations were well structured and periodic individual or group consultation was available (Kozloff, 1974; MacDonald et al., 1974).

† The Fristoe (1975) report also includes a directory of agencies offering speech, language, and hearing services in the United States.

velopment. There simply are not enough professionals to go around; especially professionals trained specially to work with the multiply or severely handicapped. Even if there were enough professionals, it would be uneconomical and inefficient to rely entirely on them for every phase of service delivery (Sigelman and Bensberg, 1976, p. 655).

The help of aides and parents is imperative in any program devoted to twenty-four-hour instruction, such as must be the case with severely hearing impaired, deaf-blind, and profoundly retarded. One such program, employing the use of aides, has been described in some detail by Kopchick and Lloyd (1976). One of the most crucial aspects of that type of program was felt to be the selection, training, and supervision of the direct care staff; they spend a great deal more time with the clients than any other personnel do. It was felt to be important that they have "the best possible training in simultaneous communication and behavior management principles and techniques" (p. 510). Since they spend so much time, as a rule, with the handicapped child, the term supportive personnel may be a misnomer; direct care personnel may be a more proper term, but such a term has acquired some custodial connotation in institutional settings.

"More recently, a new role has emerged that is much like the attendant's role. As the trend toward deinstitutionalization has taken hold, community residences have been developed, either in the form of small foster homes for children or larger group homes and half-way houses for adults. In such programs, the foster parents or 'houseparents,' as they are often called, take primary responsibility for the care and maintenance of residents. If trained and supervised by professionals, however, they also can play an important role in training activities and function as more than parent surrogates. In residential institutions, as well as in smaller community residences, coordination between professionals and supportive personnel who supervise residents during the bulk of the day is critical" (Sigelman and Bensberg, 1976, p. 656).

Many older residential institutions function under the "medical" model in which there is a one-way directional flow of commands and aides are told what to do but have little input in the planning or decision-making. In more progressive programs, a "team" model is used, which attempts to "reduce barriers among various disciplines and between professionals and various supportive personnel, including direct-care staff, by fostering [interactional] planning, diagnosis, and treatment" (Sigelman and Bensberg, 1976, p. 660).

In one study, direct-care staff were asked to classify their facility into one of four categories: autocratic, benevolent autocratic, consultative, and participative. Most attendants saw their facility as consultative, but indicated that they would like a more important role in decision-making; one which would make them feel more like members of the participative team. They viewed their positions and roles as "pivotal" but felt that their pay, training, and input into planning were inconsistent with the amount of time they were spending—comparatively—with the children. Relative to the desirability and implementation of a participative model of service delivery, Sigelman and Bensberg (1976) suggest that "it is not enough to train supportive personnel to execute plans handed down to them by professionals; professionals must be trained to use effective supervisory styles in their interactions with supportive personnel, styles that promote effective teamwork" (p. 661).

Since the severely handicapped need much more personal attention than other exceptional children, the use of aides as a resource is most important. They make it possible for the clinician to take necessary time to plan, locate, and develop materials, and they are not as expensive as professionally trained staff. It is often possible even to use age-peers as assistants in older grades and high schools. Utilizing behavior modification and highly specific and explicit procedures, peers can be almost as effective as nonpeer supportive personnel. One advantage in using peers is that they learn that severely limited children are human and can learn and develop.

Parents

Parents are in a position to interact with the child more frequently and for longer periods of time than anyone else during the early years. They therefore have the potential of being the primary language teachers, and any form of early language intervention "not using parents as a primary resource may be at best inefficient and at worst be totally ineffective" (Lloyd, 1976). In most cases it is correct to assume that the setting and circumstances that provide the most natural learning environment for the very young child center around his mother and father and his own home (Horton, 1976). This premise is so important that some of the best preschool programs for young deaf children (e.g. Tracy Clinic, Bill Wilkerson Center) take place in clinics that have a homelike atmosphere and utilize parents during the day as partners with the clinical staff working with the children.

One advantage in having parents assist in the management of a clinic or school is that they can learn to carry out similar activities at home; this kind of home activity can facilitate carry-over of clinical training, which is probably essential if generalization of new skills to the home and community context is to be realized (Spradlin and Spradlin, 1976). Garcia (1974) found that newly learned communicative skills of the severely retarded did not generalize outside of the clinical setting and these skills had to be taught in the context in which they are to be used. Generalization was stronger if the parent taught the skills in the home than it was if nonparents taught them in the home (apparently parents serve as effective contextual cues for generalization).

One of the resources that parents can supply is a fairly rich knowledge of the child, his individual idiosyncrasies, motivations, fears, etc.; such knowledge can often be put to use in the evaluation, planning, and intervention process. Another advantage in utilizing the parents is that their participation in the clinical process usually strengthens support of the program through their increased knowledge of the goals and objectives of the program in general and in relation to the specific aims for their own child. Parents can serve as important liaisons between the clinic, the home, and the community and can do much to disseminate a positive image of the clinic (Haring and Brown, 1976).

In one program, deaf children who had received supervised parental instruction, beginning early in the first year, were compared to a deaf control group whose formal instruction did not begin until after three years of age. The early intervention group were more nearly equal in language skills to normal peer children at the time they entered kindergarten than the control group (Horton, 1976). In another study, Lovaas (1973) obtained the best overall results with autistic children when parents were used to mediate the program (in Spradlin and Spradlin, 1976).

It is becoming more and more obvious that the parent group comprises a large, often motivated, and inexpensive pool that could, with adequate training, become actively engaged in the therapeutic process.

"Agencies too often have considered the parents to be primarily in need of a therapeutic experience, to 'work through' their considerable feelings about their disabled child. While not denying the reality of those feelings, some professionals have recently responded more directly to parents' frequently expressed desire for training in specific management and teaching methods. It seems tenable that many adverse attitudes and feelings are mainly the result of daily frustrations and failures in coping with a retarded child's behavior, and that as parents become more competent as teachers, psychological benefits unobtainable through just talking might ensue" (Baker and Heifetz, 1976, pp. 351-352).

Involvement of the parent as an extension of the clinician in carrying out the intervention strategies will mean that considerably more time will need to be spent with the parent, especially initially, than traditionally has been the case. Clinicians must come to realize and take into consideration individual differences among parents relative to their educational background, feelings of adequacy and confidence, personal and family problems, etc. Some parents may feel that it is too much of an extra load for them to undertake additional clinical responsibilities or that it is unfair and discriminating that they are asked to take on extra chores when parents of normal children do not have to do so (Spradlin and Spradlin, 1976). Many parents are so tied down with their child that they are seeking relief, not additional work. Most, however, will welcome involvement in the clinical process and will assume responsibilities to the extent that they are able.

It appears that the most effective way for parents to assume clinical responsibilities is to be instructed in responsive teaching techniques—behavior modification techniques tend to maximize objectivity and minimize subjectivity in the parent-child relationship. Application of behavior modification focuses parental attention on observable behaviors "and places primary concern with environmental determinants" (Baker et al., 1976, p. 352).

One example of extreme use of parents is the Portage Project in Wisconsin. It operates administratively as a regional education agency and serves twenty-three school districts in south-central rural Wisconsin. It serves 150 children between birth and six years of age, or up to the time school readiness occurs.

All instruction takes place in each child's home and the teaching is done by the parents. A home teacher is assigned to each child and family. The teacher visits each of fifteen families one day per week for 1.5 hours. An individualized curriculum is prescribed weekly based on the assessment of each child's present behaviors in the areas of language, self-help, cognitive, motor, and socialization skills. Utilizing the parents as the teacher, the Portage Project follows the precision teaching of Lindsley (1968):
1. At least three *behaviors are targeted* for learning each week. The behaviors and criteria are chosen with the goal that the child (thus the parent) will achieve success in one week.
2. *Baseline data are recorded* by the home teacher on each new task before instruction as an additional check on readiness.
3. During the week the parents implement the *actual teaching process itself*, which includes reinforcing desired behaviors and reducing or extinguishing those behaviors that interfere with learning appropriate skills.
4. The home teacher *records post-baseline data* one week later to determine if the prescribed behaviors taught by the parents have in fact been learned by the child (Shearer and Shearer, 1976, pp. 336–337).

Thus the Portage Project utilizes and trains parents in the same way that a school would use aides. Parents are shown what to teach, how to teach, and how to observe and record behavior. Although this program perhaps puts a burden on the parents, the instigators feel that there are some unique advantages: (1) learning occurs in the parent and child's natural environment; (2) the home provides direct and constant access to behavior as it occurs naturally; (3) learned behavior will generalize and be maintained; (4) there is more opportunity for full family participation in the teaching process; (5) access is provided to the full range of behaviors; (6) training of parents will provide them with the skills necessary to deal with new behaviors when they occur; and (7) individualization of instructional goals is an operational reality (Shearer and Shearer, 1976, p. 337).

Active and enlightened parent participation with the handicapped child during the first three or four years of his life is considered to be very important. "The child at this early age is not amenable to a typical child-oriented instruction program even as informal as the nursery-kindergarten class usually is. It is the parents, the child's natural teachers, to whom one must turn. By focusing efforts on the parents and teaching them to capitalize on the innumerable ways in which auditory and language learning can occur on a daily basis in the child's home setting, the child can best be helped" (Horton, 1976, p. 374).

Two current parent-oriented preprepared training manuals for overall training are CAMS (Casto, 1977) and the Read Project Series (Baker et al., 1973, 1976). The basic notion behind preprepared programs is that they provide tailor-made procedures to meet the needs of the child and minimize the need for parents to make independent professional judgments.

Baker and Heifetz (1976) found that parents could learn to teach specific self-help skills by use of self-contained instructional packages about as well as those who received face-to-face training from the clinician; instructional packages, however, were not as effective in helping parents eradicate maladaptive behavior (p. 366). In order to make intervention by parents maximally effective, they should be able to participate in the selection of goals or objectives to be worked with (Spradlin and Spradlin, 1976).

SUMMARY

The present chapter has presented a frame of reference emphasizing the role of the clinical-specialist as a resource person to those who are responsible for the severely handicapped person's direct care. As a member of the team of specialists involved in individual evaluation, planning, and providing intervention strategies, the speech pathologist must broaden his capacity to synthesize programming of language and communication objectives with the various other specialized services in order to help maintain a more meaningful relationship in an "interdisciplinary" approach to training.

LANGUAGE OBJECTIVES* FROM INGRAM AND EISENSON (1972)†

LEVEL I: AVERAGE UTTERANCE RANGE 2.0-2.5 WORDS

Basic Constructions

1. Verb + noun,
   e.g. eat cookie
2. Adjective + noun,
   e.g. little dog.
3. Possessor + noun,
   e.g. Tom ('s) ball.
4. Noun + verb,
   e.g. boy run.

5. Noun + predicate adjective,
   e.g. boy (is) tall.
6. *That* + predicate noun,
   e.g. that (is a) ball.
7. Noun + *here, there,*
   (as locatives),
   e.g. boy (is) here; girl (is)
   there.

Function Words

1. Prepositions

   a. *In* + noun,
      e.g. in (the) box.
   b. Verb + preposition +
      noun,
      e.g. put in the box.
   c. Preposition + adjective
      + noun,
      e.g. in big truck.

   d. Preposition + possessive
      + noun,
      e.g. in John ('s) truck.
   e. Noun + *here, there,*
      e.g. ball in there.
   f. *That* + *here, there* (as
      locatives),
      e.g. that in there.

2. Pronouns

   a. Verb + *it,*
      e.g. eat it.
   b. Verb + *me,*
      e.g. carry me.
   c. *It* + verb,
      e.g. it fall (s).

   d. *I* + verb,
      e.g. I walk.
   e. *My* + noun,
      e.g. my ball.
   f. *My* + adjective + noun,
      e.g. my big ball.

---

* Parenthesis render component optional.

† Abridged and adapted from J. Eisenson, *Aphasia in Children* (© by Jon Eisenson), 1972, pp. 153-168. Courtesy of Harper & Row Pubs., Inc., New York.

g. *It + here, there* (as locatives), e.g. it here

h. *You +* verb, e.g. you walk.

3. Verb + particle, e.g. fall down

4. Noun + verb + particle, e.g. boy fall down.

Combinations of Above Forms

1. Verb + *in* + *it,* e.g. go in it.
2. Verb + *in* + adjective + noun, e.g. go in little box.
3. Verb + *in,* possessor + noun, e.g. put in Bobby truck.

4. Verb + *in* + *my* + noun, e.g. put in my box.
5. Verb + *in* + *here, there,* e.g. go in there.
6. *I +* verb + particle, e.g. I fall down.
7. *It +* verb + particle, e.g. it go (goes) up.

LEVEL II: AVERAGE UTTERANCE RANGE 2.5-3.0 WORDS

Basic Constructions

1. Noun + verb + noun, e.g. boy hit ball.
2. Verb + adjective + noun, e.g. eat big cookie.

3. Verb + possessor + noun, e.g. eat Tom (Tom's) cookie.

Function Words

1. *This, that* (demonstratives)
   a. *This, that* + predicate noun, e.g. this (is a) ball.

   b. *This, that* + predicate adjective, e.g. this green.

2. Preposition *on*
   a. *On +* noun, e.g. on table.
   b. Verb + *on* + noun, e.g. put on table.

   c. *On +* adjective + noun, e.g. on big table.
   d. Noun + verb + *on* + noun, e.g. Bobby sit on chair.

3. Articles
   a. *A* + noun,
      e.g. a cat.
   b. *The* + noun,
      e.g. the cat.
   c. Verb + article + noun,
      e.g. get a ball.
   d. Noun + verb + article
      + noun,
      e.g. boy eat a cookie.
   e. Article + adjective +
      noun,
      e.g. a big ball.

4. Inflections
   a. Plurals
      (1) Nouns,
          e.g. boys.
      (2) Verb + noun,
          e.g. see birds.
      (3) Noun + verb +
          noun,
          e.g. boy see car.
   b. Progressive form
      (1) Noun + verb,
          e.g. boy running.
      (2) Noun + verb +
          noun,
          e.g. man driving car.

Combinations of Above Forms

1. Noun + verb + *in* + noun,
   e.g. Tom put in box.
2. Noun + preposition +
   noun,
   e.g. ball in box.
3. Verb + preposition +
   adjective + noun,
   e.g. put in big box.
4. Verb + preposition +
   possessor + noun,
   e.g. put in Tom box.
5. Noun + verb + *it*,
   e.g. girl take it.
6. Noun +verb + *me*,
   e.g. girl push me.
7. *It* + verb + noun,
   e.g. it go home.
8. *I* + verb + noun,
   e.g. I catch ball.
9. *You* + verb + noun,
   e.g. you catch ball.
10. Verb + *my* + noun,
    e.g. hold my doll.
11. Progressive verb + plural
    noun,
    e.g. putting blocks.
12. Noun + progressive verb
    + plural noun,
    e.g. boy putting blocks.
13. Progressive verb + article
    + noun,
    e.g. eating a cookie.

Question Forms

1. *What*

    a. What that?

    b. What boy do?

    c. What boy read?

    d. What boy ('s) name?

2. *Where*

    a. Where ('s) that?

    b. Where girl go?

    c. Where boy run?

LEVEL III: AVERAGE UTTERANCE RANGE 3.0-4.0 WORDS

Basic Constructions

1. Noun + verb + noun,
   e.g. man open door.
2. Verb + noun + preposition,
   e.g. put in box.
3. Modal + verb + noun,
   e.g. going play ball.
4. Noun + verb + noun +
   preposition phrase,
   e.g. boy put ball in box.
5. Noun + copula + noun,
   e.g. doll is (a) girl.
6. Demonstrative + *is* + noun,
   e.g. that is boy.
7. Noun + *is* + *here, there,*
   e.g. dog is there.
8. Noun + *is* + *in, on* + noun,
   e.g. dog is in box.
9. Noun + *is* + predicate
   adjective,
   e.g. ball is red.

Function Words

1. Plural inflections,
   e.g. put balls in box.
2. Progressive,
   e.g. boy is running.
3. Articles, *a, the,*
   e.g. put a block in box.
4. Conjunction *and,*
   e.g. boy and girl.
5. Preposition *at, to,*
   e.g. at school; boy at school;
   go to school; girl is at store;
   boy go to school.
6. Pronouns *she, he, him, her,*
   them, their,
   e.g. she throw ball; he chase
   her; she is their; he is at
   school; she gonna eat cookie;
   he put them in; they get in
   wagon; she give cookie to
   him.

Combination of Above Forms

1. Noun + modal + verb +
   prepositional phrase,
   e.g. boy gonna go to store.
2. Pronoun + verb +
   progressive,
   e.g. he is running.
3. Noun + progressive + verb
   + prepositional phrase,
   e.g. dog is running to boy.
4. Pronoun + verb + plural
   noun,
   e.g. he eats cookies.

Question Forms

1. *What, where,*
   e.g. What is that?
   Where is the girl going?
2. Yes or no question with
   inverted *is.*
   a. Noun + copula +noun,
      e.g. Is Rover (a) dog?
   b. Noun + copula +
      preposition + noun,
      e.g. Is dog in box?
   c. Noun + copula +
      progressive verb,
      e.g. Is dog barking?
3. Tag question,
   e.g. I put ball in box, OK?

NONVOCAL APPROACHES TO LANGUAGE COMMUNICATION

THIS ADDENDUM briefly describes various nonvocal systems that are frequently being used as alternative systems for children who do not respond adequately to vocal language-communication training. It is impractical to attempt to describe all available systems; only those more commonly in use are discussed here.

Sign Language Systems

American Sign Language (AMESLAN) is a formalized version of the older form of manual signing in the United States (Fant, 1972) and is used by the majority of deaf adults (Wilbur, 1976). This system is not correlated with the English syntax and recently an English syntax form of signing (Signed English) has been developed and has become very popular for use in teaching sign language to young children. Signed English uses manual symbols (symbols made with the hands) adopted mainly from the American Sign Language, but also draws from other systems developed in the United States, such as Signing Exact English, Seeing Essential English, and Linguistics of Visual English (Bornstein, 1974; Bornstein et al., 1975).

The greatest advantage of Signed English is that it utilizes exact English syntax and therefore it can be signed and spoken in synchrony; this facilitates using a more total communication approach, i.e. teaching the manual and spoken forms of the language simultaneously. For this reason this system seems to be appropriate for nonvocal handicapped children for whom a visual signing system may have a facilitating influence on the development of vocal symbols.

A dictionary developed at Gallaudet College for use with very young children lists a basic vocabulary of over 2,000 words that various research studies indicated were most frequently heard and used by normal preschool children (Bornstein et al., 1975).

Most of the signs (1,353) used for these words were taken from the American Sign Language (AMESLAN); the others were taken from other signing sources. Special sign markers are given that represent certain aspects of English syntax such as verb tenses, adverbs, adjectives, plural, person, possessive, comparative, agent, contractions, compounds, etc.

This dictionary does not illustrate any sentence construction, but a series of booklets, also available through Gallaudet College Press, can be used by parents and others to teach words and their use in sentences. These booklets emphasize beginning books such as *Baby Animal Book, My Toy Book;* stories or poems such as *Little Red Riding Hood, Three Little Kittens;* and growing up books such as *I Want to Be a Farmer, We're Going to the Doctor.* Current lists and prices on these materials can be obtained by writing to Gallaudet College Press.

Another excellent resource for clinicians or other trainees learning and teaching a basic signing repertoire is a series of films, both projector type and portable hand-cranked viewer type (Huffman et al., 1975). These films are relatively inexpensive (especially the hand-cranked viewer types) and have the advantage of a moving model of words and phrases along with a written caption for easy learning. The words and sentences in these films are clustered together in terms of functional classifications—for example, family and friends, emotions and feelings, what-we-do, body parts, colors and numbers, clothing, grooming, at-the-table, around-the-house, time, animals, transportation, etc.—with a separate film cartridge for each category. This package of materials has a 400 word vocabulary adopted for use with severely handicapped children by the California State Department of Health.

An introductory programmed text by O'Rourke (1973) gives signs and exercises for a fairly basic adult vocabulary and has an annotated bibliography of various resources and media that can be utilized in the learning and teaching of sign language.

For an excellent list of studies and reports on the use of manual communication as a nonverbal alternative to vocal language training, the reader may wish to obtain Fristoe and Lloyd's

(1977) article that lists a comprehensive bibliography on this subject.

Bliss Symbolics

The Bliss symbols were developed by Bliss (1965) between 1942 and 1949. They were inspired by Chinese pictographic writing and the desire for a common world system for communication. Use of Bliss symbolics with severely handicapped began in 1971 at the Ontario Crippled Children's Center, primarily with children who had cerebral palsy. By 1974 over sixty programs throughout the United States were using Bliss symbolics as one of their nonvocal alternatives with severely handicapped.

There are 100 basic elements in this system and variations in number, size, and position enable the generation of an infinite number of symbols; therefore, symbols have to be drawn to a particular scale. Each symbol represents a visual concept rather than a single word, which may be one reason why severely handicapped can learn them with relative ease. Tense, plurals, questions, negatives, etc., are represented by specific symbol markers.

The beginning program uses a lapboard with 100 basic symbols already drawn and arranged into vertical categories. The written word is printed under each symbol; thus anyone who can read can interpret the symbol (see Figure 4). The child indicates the symbol of his choice, or combination of symbols for more complex ideas, by pointing to it (them) on the board. The more advanced programs have a 200 word chart and a 400 word chart, each of which can be used as a lapboard.

The suggested requisites for the child's being able to respond to the Bliss symbol program (Harris-Vanderheiden, 1976) are the following: (1) must be able to establish eye contact, (2) must demonstrate knowledge of object permanence, (3) must be able to attend to a task for a five-minute period, (4) must be able to follow auditory directions, and (5) must have a desire to communicate. A number of articles describe for the clinician who is not very familiar with this system how it can best be used with severely handicapped children (Harris-Vanderheiden et al., 1975; Harris-Vanderheiden, 1976; McNaughton, 1976; Archer, 1977).*

---

* Materials and instructions can be ordered from Blissymbolics Communication Foundation, 862 Eglinton Avenue East, Toronto, Canada, MHG 211.

	a	b	c	d	e	f	g	h	i	j	
1	0	1	2	3	4	5	6	7	8	9	1
2	hello ⟲ good-bye	[?] question	1₁ I,me(my)	♡+! like	♡↑ happy	make action	food	pen,pencil	1♡+! friend	animal	2
3	!♡ please	?▷ why	1₂ you(your)	♡? want	x♡≪ angry	mouth	drink	paper, page	GOD	bird	3
4	♡⚓ thanks	?∧ how	man	→| come	♡!? afraid	eye	sleep	book	house	flower	4
5	I'm sorry	?! who	woman	give	♡↑o funny	legs	toilet	table	school	water	5
6	opposite	?□ what thing	father	make	good	hand	pain	television	hospital	sun	6
7	much, many	?÷ which	mother	help	big	ear	clothing	news	store	weather	7
8	music	where	brother	think	young,new	nose	outing	word	show	day	8
9		when	sister	know	difficult	head	car	light	room	week-end	9
10		?x how many	teacher	wash	hot	name	wheelchair	game,toy	street	birthday	10
	a	b	c	d	e	f	g	h	i	j	

Figure 4. 100 Blissymbol display board, December 1975. © Blissymbolics Communication Institute. Blissymbols used herein C. K. Bliss and exclusive worldwide licensee B.C.I., Toronto, Canada.

Communication Boards

Vanderheiden (1976) and his colleagues at the Trace Research and Development Center at the University of Wisconsin have described three general types of communication boards for use with nonvocal communicatively handicapped. These approaches are designed to compensate for lack of vocal communication as well as for various types of physical disability. All three approaches utilize the same basic components: (1) physical means of indicating, (2) symbol system, and (3) rules for generating a variety of meaningful symbol combinations.

Three general methods of communication utilizing nonvocal procedures include *scanning, encoding,* and *direct selection.*

Boards have been classified in accordance with the type of communicating method that they facilitate (Vanderheiden, 1976).

SCANNING BOARDS. In this approach, the spectator (or an electronic or mechanical device) scans a large sample of symbols and the child indicates "yes" or "no" to identify the symbols he wishes to communicate. "The simplest example of a scanning technique would be the familiar 'yes/no' guessing [20 questions] technique. . . . Another example of a simple scanning technique would be the use of a communication board with a second person pointing to the pictures, words, or letters one at a time while watching for a response from the child" (Vanderheiden, 1976, pp. 21-22). The first column of Figure 5 illustrates various types of scanning procedures.

CLASSIFICATION TYPE

		1. Scanning	2. Encoding	3. Direct Selection
	Unaided			
LEVEL OF IMPLEMENTATION	Fundamental			
	Simple Electronic			
	Fully Independent (Printed Output)			
	Fully Independent and Portable			

Figure 5. Examples of techniques for providing various forms of nonvocal communication. From Gregg C. Vanderheiden and Kate Grilley, *Non-vocal Communication Techniques and Aids for the Severely Physically Handicapped,* p. 28. © 1976 University Park Press, Baltimore, Maryland.

ENCODING BOARDS. A simplified example of the encoding approach to indicating symbolically is the method routinely utilized for locating positions on a map. A board displaying any number of symbols (such as those in Figure 4) may utilize an array of indicator-codes along the vertical (ordinate) and horizontal (abscissa) margins; any single cell on the display can be located precisely by indicating the appropriate marginal codes. The second column of Figure 5 illustrates various levels of encoding devices.

DIRECT SELECTION BOARDS. This method may be used most efficiently by children with fairly good visual-motor and manual skills, since it employs some means of directly indicating the symbol or message to be conveyed. This type of board is perhaps the most commonly used nonvocal form of communication. The third column of Figure 5 illustrates various levels of direct selection devices.

References

Archer, L. A.: Blissymbolics—A nonverbal communication system. *J Speech Hear Disord, 42:*568-579, 1977.

Azrin, N. H., Bugle, C. P., and O'Brien, F.: Behavioral engineering: Two apparatuses for toilet training retarded children. *J Appl Behav Anal, 4:*249-253, 1971.

Baer, D. M., Peterson, R. F., and Sherman, J. A.: The development of imitation by reinforcing behavior similarity to a model. *J Exp Anal Behav, 10:* 405-416, 1967.

Baker, B. L., Brightman, A. J., Heifetz, L. J., and Murphy, D. M.: *Read project series: 10 instructional manuals for parents.* Cambridge, Massachusetts: Behavioral Education Projects, 1973.

Baker, B. L., Brightman, A. J., Heifetz, L. J., and Murphy, D. M.: *Steps to independence series.* Champaign, Illinois: Res Press, 1976.

Baker, B. L. and Heifetz, L. J.: The Read project: Teaching manuals for parents of retarded children. In Tjossem, T. D. (Ed.): *Intervention strategies for high risk infants and young children.* Baltimore, Maryland: Univ Park, 1976.

Bartin, E. S., Guess, D., Garcia, E., and Baer, D. M.: Improvements of retardates' mealtime behaviors by timeout procedures using multiple baseline techniques. *J Appl Behav Anal, 3:*77-84, 1970.

Berry, M. F.: *Language disorders of children: The bases and diagnoses.* New York: Appleton-Century-Crofts, 1969.

Bliss, C. K.: *Semantography.* Sydney, Australia: Semantography Publications, 1965.

Bornstein, H.: Signed English: A manual approach to English language development. *J Speech Hear Disord, 39*:330-343, 1974.

Bornstein, H., Hamilton, L. B., Saulnier, K. L., and Roy, H. L. (Eds.): *The signed English dictionary for preschool and elementary levels.* Washington, D.C.: Gallaudet College Press, 1975.

Breland, M.: Application of method. In Bensberg, G. J. (Ed.): *Teaching mentally retarded children.* Atlanta, Georgia: Southern Regional Educational Board, 1965.

Bricker, D. D.: Imitative sign training as a facilitator of word-object association with low functioning children. *Am J Ment Defic, 76*:509-516, 1972.

Bricker, D. D.: Educational synthesizer. In Thomas, M. A. (Ed.): *Hey, don't forget about me!* Reston, Virginia: Council for Exceptional Children, 1976.

Bricker, W. A. and Bricker, D. D.: A program of language training for the severely language handicapped child. *Except Child, 37*:101-111, 1970.

Bricker, W. A. and Bricker, D. D.: An early language training strategy. Schiefelbusch, R. L. (Ed.): *Language perspectives: Acquisition, retardation, and intervention.* Baltimore, Maryland: Univ Park, 1974.

Bricker, W. A. and Bricker, D. D.: The infant toddler and preschool research and intervention project. In Tjossem, T. D. (Ed.): *Intervention strategies for high risk infants and young children.* Baltimore, Maryland: Univ Park, 1976.

Bricker, D., Dennison, L., Watson, L., and Vincent-Smith, L.: *Language training program for young developmentally delayed children.* IMRID Behavioral Science Monograph 22, Nashville, Tenn.: Institute on Mental Retardation and Intellectual Development, George Peabody College, 1973.

Bricker, D. D., Ruder, K. F., and Vincent, L.: An intervention strategy for language deficient children. In Haring, N. G. and Schiefelbusch, R. L. (Eds.): *Teaching special children.* New York: McGraw, 1976.

Buros, O. K.: The seventh mental measurements yearbook. Highland Park, New Jersey: Gryphon Pr NJ, 1972.

Carrier, J. K.: Application of functional analysis and a non-speech response mode to teaching language (Parsons Research Center Report No. 7). Parsons, Kansas: Parsons State Hospital and Training Center, 1973.

Carrier, J. K. and Peak, T.: *Non-speech language initiation program.* Lawrence, Kansas: H and H Enterprises, 1975.

Carrier, J. K.: Application of a nonspeech language system with the severely language handicapped. In Lloyd, L. L. (Ed.): *Communication assessment intervention strategies.* Baltimore, Maryland: Univ Park, 1976.

Casto, G. (Ed.): *Curriculum and monitoring system (CAMS).* Logan, Utah: Utah State University Exceptional Child Center, 1977.

Ciminero, A. R.: Behavioral assessment: An overview. In Ciminero, A. R., Calhoun, K. S., and Adams, H. E. (Eds.): *Handbook of behavioral assessment.* New York: Wiley, 1977.

Cheney, C. and Kephart, N. M.: *Motoric aids to perceptual learning.* Columbus, Ohio: Merrill, 1968.

Cody, W. J. and Borkowski, J. G.: Proactive interference and its release in short-term memory of mildly retarded adolescents. *Am J Ment Defic, 82:* 305-308, 1977.

Connell, P. J., Spradlin, J. E., and McReynolds, L. V.: Some suggested criteria for evaluating of language programs. *J Speech Hear Disord, 42:*563-567, 1977.

Cratty, B. J.: *Perceptual-motor behavior and educational processes.* Springfield: Thomas, 1968.

Cratty, B. J.: The use of movement activities in the education of retarded children. In Pearson, P. H. and Williams, C. E. (Eds.): *Physical therapy services in the developmental disabilities.* Springfield: Thomas, 1972.

Creedon, M. P. (Ed.): Appropriate behavior through communication; A new program in simultaneous language for nonverbal children (unpublished manual). Dysfunctioning Child Center, Michael Reese Medical Center, Chicago, Illinois, 1974.

Darley, F. L., Siegel, G. M., Fay, W. M., Newman, P. W., and Rees, M. (Eds.): *Evaluation of assessment techniques in speech pathology.* New York: A-W, in press.

Diedrich, W. M.: *Charting speech behavior.* Kansas City, Kansas: Extramural Independent Study Center, University of Kansas, 1973.

Eisenson, J.: *Aphasia in children.* New York: Har-Row, 1972.

Fant, L. J., Jr.: *Ameslan.* Silver Spring, Maryland: Nat Assn Deaf, 1972.

Finnie, N.: *Handling the young cerebral palsied child at home.* London: Heinemann, 1970.

Flavell, J. H.: Developmental studies in mediated memory. In Reese, H. W. and Lipsitt, L. D. (Eds.): *Advances in child development and behavior,* vol. 5. New York: Acad Pr, 1970.

Foxx, R. M. and Azrin, N. H.: The elimination of autistic self-stimulation behavior by overcorrection. *J Appl Behav Analysis, 6:*1-14, 1973.

Fristoe, M.: Language intervention systems for the retarded. Montgomery, Alabama: State of Alabama Department of Education, 1975.

Fristoe, M.: Language intervention systems: Programs published in kit form. In Lloyd, L. L. (Ed.) *Communication assessment and intervention strategies.* Baltimore, Maryland: Univ Park, 1976.

Fristoe, M. and Lloyd, L. L.: Manual communication for the retarded and others with severe communicative impairment: A resource list. *Ment Retard, 15:*18-21, 1977.

Gallacher, J. J., Ramey, C. T., Haskins, R., and Finkelstein, N. W.: Use of longitudinal research in the study of child development. In Tjossem, T. D. (Ed.): *Intervention strategies for high risk infants and young children.* Baltimore, Maryland: Univ Park, 1976.

Garcia, E. E.: The training and generalization of a conversational speech form in nonverbal retardates. *J Appl Behav Analysis, 7:*137-151, 1974.

Gelfand, D. M. and Hartmann, D. D.: *Child behavior analysis and therapy.* New York: Pergamon, 1975.

Gentry, D. and Haring, N. G.: Essentials of performance measurement. In Haring, N. G. and Brown, L. J. (Eds.): *Teaching the severely handicapped,* vol. 1. New York: Grune and Stratton, 1976.

Gronlund, N. E.: *Constructing achievement tests.* Englewood Cliffs, N.J.: Prentice-Hall, 1977.

Haring, N. G. and Brown, L. J.: *Teaching the severely handicapped,* vol. 1. New York: Grune, 1976.

Harris-Vanderheiden, C., Brown, W. P., MacKenzie, P., Reinen, S., and Scheibel, C.: Symbol communication for the mentally handicapped: An application of Bliss symbols as an alternate communication mode for non-vocal mentally retarded children with motoric impairment. *Ment Retard, 13,* 1975.

Harris-Vanderheiden, C.: Blissymbols and the mentally retarded. In Vanderheiden, G. C. and Grilley, K. (Eds.): *Non-vocal communication technique and aids for the severely physically handicapped.* Baltimore, Maryland: Univ Park, 1976.

Hartup, W. W.: Report of the education committee. In Tjossem, T. D. (Ed.): *Intervention strategies for high risk infants and young children.* Baltimore, Maryland: Univ Park, 1976.

Henricksen, K. and Doughty, R.: Decelerating undesired mealtime behavior in a group of profoundly retarded boys. *Am J Ment Defic, 72:*40-44, 1967.

Hersen, M. and Barlow, D. H.: *Single case experimental designs: Strategies for studying behavior change.* New York: Pergamon, 1976.

Hollis, J. H.: Direct measurement of the effects of drugs and alternative activity on stereotyped behavior (Working Paper No. 168). Parsons, Kansas: Parsons State Hospital and Training Center, 1967.

Horton, K. B.: Early intervention for hearing impaired infants and young children. In Tjossem, T. D. (Ed.): *Intervention strategies for high risk infants and young children.* Baltimore, Maryland: Univ Park, 1976.

Huffman, J., Hoffman, B., Gransee, D., Fox, A., James, J., and Schmitz, J.: *Talk with me: Communication with the multihandicapped deaf.* Northridge, California: Joyce Motion Picture Co., 1975.

Hughs, J.: Language and communication: acquisition of a non-vocal "language" by previously languageless children. Unpublished bachelor of technology thesis, Brunel University, 1972.

Ingram, D. and Eisenson, J.: Therapeutic approaches III: Establishing and developing language in congenitally aphasic children. In Eisenson, J.: *Aphasia in children.* New York: Har-Row, 1972.

Jackson, S. E.: Individualized instruction. In Taylor, G. R. and Jackson, S. E. (Eds.): *Educational strategies and services for exceptional children.* Springfield: Thomas, 1976.

Jackson, S. E., Lattimore, I., Hawkins, C., and Jones, R.: Organizational in-structural strategies. In Taylor, G. R. and Jackson, S. E. (Eds.): *Educational strategies and services for exceptional children.* Springfield: Thomas, 1976.

Johnson, D. J. and Myklebust, H. R.: *Learning disabilities.* New York: Grune, 1967.

Johnson, N. F.: Chunking and the organization of behavior. In Bower, G. H. (Ed.): *The psychology of learning and motivation.* New York: Acad Pr, 1970.

Jones, J. D.: Sensory motor treatment for severe and profoundly retarded children. In Kramer, K. F. and Rosonke, R. (Eds.): *State of the art: Diagnosis and treatment.* Reston, Virginia: National Resource Center Conference Report, 1974.

Jones, J. D.: Sensory-motor training of the severely handicapped. Paper presented to the American Association for the Education of the Severely/Profoundly Handicapped, Baltimore, Maryland, 1978.

Kahn, J. V.: A comparison of manual and oral training with mute retarded children. *Ment Retard, 15:*21-23, 1977.

Kent, L. R.: A language acquisition program for the retarded. In McLean, J. E., Yoder, D. E., and Schiefelbusch, R. L. (Eds.): *Language intervention with the retarded: Developing strategies.* Boston, Massachusetts: Univ Park, 1972.

Kent, L. R.: *Language acquisition program for the severely retarded.* Champaign, Illinois: Res Press, 1974.

Kent, R. N. and Foster, S. L.: Direct observational procedures: Methodological issues in naturalistic settings. In Ciminero, A. R., Calhoun, K. S., and Adams, H. E. (Eds.): *Handbook of behavioral assessment.* New York: Wiley, 1977.

Kopchick, G. A. and Lloyd, L. L.: Total communication for the severely language impaired: A 24-hour approach. In Lloyd, L. L. (Ed.): *Communication assessment and intervention strategies.* Baltimore, Maryland: Univ Park, 1976.

Kozloff, M.: Parents as teachers. *Forum, 15:*8-12, 1974.

Leonard, L. R.: Relational meaning and the facilitation of slow-learning children's language. *Am J Ment Defic, 80:*180-185, 1975.

Lloyd, L. L.: Discussant's comments: Language and communication aspects. In Tjossem, T. D. (Ed.): *Intervention strategies for high risk infants and young children.* Baltimore, Maryland: Univ Park, 1976.

Loftus, G. R. and Loftus, E. F.: *Human memory: The processing of information.* New York: Wiley, 1976.

Lovaas, O. I. and Simmons, J. Q.: Manipulation of self-destruction in three retarded children. *J Appl Behav Analysis, 2:*143-159, 1969.

Luria, A. R.: *Cognitive development: Its cultural and social foundations.* Cambridge, Massachusetts: Harvard U Pr, 1976.

MacDonald, J. D., Blott, J. P., Gordon, K., Spiegel, B., and Hartmann, M.:

An experimental parent-assisted treatment program for pre-school language delayed children. *J Speech Hear Disord, 39:*395-415, 1974.

Maharaj, S. C.: *Language sequence program.* Moose Jaw, Saskatchewan, Canada: Valley View Center (Department of Speech and Hearing), 1975.

Mahoney, K., Van Wagenen, R. K., and Meyerson, L.: Toilet training of normal and retarded children. *J Appl Behav Analysis, 4:*173-183, 1971.

McNaughton, S.: Bliss symbols—an alternative symbol system for the nonvocal pre-reading child. In Vanderheiden, G. C. and Grilley, K. (Eds.): *Non-vocal communication techniques and aids for the severely hand capped.* Baltimore, Maryland: Univ Park, 1976.

McNeill, D.: *The acquisition of language: The study of developmental psycholinguistics.* New York: Har-Row, 1970.

Mecham, M. J.: *Development of audiolinguistic skills in children.* St. Louis, Missouri: Green, 1969.

Mecham, M. J.: *Motivation and learning-centered training programs for language delayed children.* Salt Lake City, Utah: Wordmaking Productions, 1977.

Mecham, M. J.: Attentional disturbances and their implications in early language intervention with severely handicapped children. Paper presented to the American Association for the Education of the Severely/Profoundly Handicapped, Baltimore, Maryland, 1978.

Menyuk, P.: Syntactic structures in the language of children. *Child Dev, 34:* 407-422, 1963.

Miller, G. A.: The magical number seven, plus or minus two: Some limits on our capacity to process information. *Psychol Rev, 63:*81-97, 1956.

Miller, J. F. and Yoder, D. E.: An ontogenetic language teaching strategy for retarded children. In Schiefelbusch, R. L. (Ed.): *Language perspectives: Acquisition, retardation, and intervention.* Baltimore, Maryland: Univ Park, 1974.

Morehead, D. M. and Morehead, A.: From signal to sign: A piagetian view of thought and language during the first two years. In Schiefelbusch, R. L. (Ed.): *Language perspectives—Acquisition, retardation, and intervention.* Baltimore, Maryland: Univ Park, 1974.

Morehead, D. M. and Morehead, A. E. (Eds.): *Normal and deficient child language.* Baltimore, Maryland: Univ Park, 1976.

Mowrer, D.: *Developing precision in recording speech behaviors.* Salt Lake City, Utah: Word Making Productions, 1971.

Murdock, J. and Hartmann, B.: *A language development program: Imitative gestures to basic syntactic structures.* Salt Lake City, Utah: Wordmaking Productions, 1975.

O'Brien, F., Bugle, C., and Azrin, N. H.: Training and maintaining a retarded child's proper eating. *J Appl Behav Analysis, 5:*67-73, 1972.

Ontario Crippled Children's Center: *Teaching guide, symbol communication project.* Toronto, Canada: Ontario Crippled Children's Center, 1974.

O'Rourke, T. J.: *A basic course in manual communication.* Washington, D.C.: National Association for the Deaf, 1973.

Peter, L. J.: *Competencies for teaching individual instruction.* Belmont, California: Wadsworth Pub, 1975.

Piaget, J.: *The Child and Reality.* New York: Grossman Publishers, 1973.

Popovich, D.: *A prescriptive behavioral checklist for the severely and profoundly retarded.* Baltimore, Maryland: University Park Press, 1977.

Prouty, R. and Prillaman, D.: *Diagnostic teaching: A modest proposal. Elementary School Journal,* 70:265-270, 1970.

Reagan, C. L.: *Handbook of auditory perceptual training.* Springfield: Thomas, 1973.

Reger, R.: *Preschool programming of children with disabilities.* Springfield: Thomas, 1970.

Reichart, G. J., Cody, W. J., and Borkowski, J. G.: Training and transfer of clustering and cumulative rehearsal strategies in retarded individuals. *Am J Ment Defic,* 79:648-658, 1975.

Richardson, T.: Sign language for SMR and PMR. *Ment Retard,* 13:17, 1975.

Rogers, C. R.: *Client-centered therapy.* Boston, Massachusetts: HM, 1951.

Schiefelbusch, R. L. and Haring, N. G.: Perspectives on teaching special children. In Haring, N. G. and Schiefelbusch, R. L. (Eds.): *Teaching special children.* New York: McGraw, 1976.

Schiefelbusch, R. L., Ruder, K. F., and Bricker, W. A.: Training strategies for language-deficient children: An overview. In Haring, N. G. and Schiefelbusch, R. L. (Eds.): *Teaching special children.* New York: McGraw, 1976.

Shaffer, T. R. and Goehl, H.: The alinguistic child. *Ment Retard,* 12:3-6, 1974.

Shearer, D. E. and Shearer, M. S.: The Portage Project: A model for early childhood intervention. In Tjossem, T. D. (Ed.): *Intervention strategies for high risk infants and young children.* Baltimore, Maryland: Univ Park, 1976.

Sigelman, C. K. and Bensberg, G. J.: Supportive personnel for the developmentally disabled. In Lloyd, L. L. (Ed.): *Communication assessment and intervention strategies.* Baltimore, Maryland: Univ Park, 1976.

Spradlin, J. E.: The Premack hypothesis and self-feeding by profoundly retarded children: A case report. Parsons, Kansas: Parsons State Hospital and Training Center (Parsons Working Paper No. 79), 1964.

Spradlin, J. E., Girardeau, F. L., and Corte, E.: Fixed ratio and fixed interval behavior of behavior of severely and profoundly retarded subjects. *J Exp Child Psychol,* 2:340-353, 1966.

Spradlin, J. E. and Spradlin, R. R.: Developing necessary skills for entry into classroom teaching arrangements. In Haring, N. G. and Schiefelbusch, R. L. (Eds.): *Teaching special children.* New York: McGraw, 1976.

Taylor, G. R. and Jackson, S. E.: *Educational strategies and services for exceptional children*. Springfield: Thomas, 1976.

Topper, S. T.: Gesture language for a non-verbal severely retarded male. *Ment Retard, 13*:30-31, 1975.

Utley, J.: *What's its name?* Urbana, Illinois: U of Ill Pr, 1950.

Valetutti, P. and Grosman, J. F.: *College and university programs*. In Taylor, G. R. and Jackson, S. E. (Eds.): *Educational strategies and services for exceptional children*. Springfield: Thomas, 1976.

Vanderheiden, G. C.: Providing the child with a means to indicate. In Vanderheiden, G. C. and Grilley, K. (Eds.): *Non-vocal communication techniques and aids for the severely physically handicapped*. Baltimore, Maryland: Univ Park, 1976.

Vanderheiden, G. C. and Grilley, K.: *Non-vocal communication techniques and aids for the severely physically handicapped*. Baltimore, Maryland: Univ Park, 1976.

Vygotsky, L.: *Thought and language*. Cambridge, Massachusetts: MIT Pr, 1962.

White, O. R. and Liberty, K. A.: Behavioral assessment and precise educational measurement. In Haring, N. G. and Schiefelbusch, R. L. (Eds.): *Teaching special children*. New York: McGraw, 1976.

Whitney, L. R. and Barnard, K. E.: Implications of operant learning theory for nursing care of the retarded child. *Ment Retard, 4*:26-29, 1966.

Wickens, D. D.: Characteristics of word encoding. In Melton, A. W. and Martin, E. (Eds.) *Coding processes in human memory*. Washington, D.C.: Winston, 1972.

Wilbur, R. B.: The linguistics of manual languages and manual systems. In Lloyd, L. L. (Ed.): *Communication assessment and intervention and assessment strategies*. Baltimore, Maryland: Univ Park, 1976.

Wilhelm, H. and Lovaas, O. I.: Stimulus over-selectivity: A common feature in autism and mental retardation. *Am J Ment Defic, 81*:18-25, 1976.

Wilson, P. S.: Sign language as a means of communication for the mentally retarded. Paper presented at the Eastern Psychological Association meeting, Philadelphia, Pennsylvania, 1974.

AUTHOR INDEX

SUBJECT INDEX

A

Abstracting, 243
Ameslan, 272, 273
Analysis of spontaneous sample, 173-176
Assembly *vs* differentiation, *See* developmental issues
Assessment in Infancy, 114-161
Assessment of Children's Language Comprehension, 118
Attentional deficits, 73-74
Auditory figure-ground differentiation, 241

B

Bankson Language Screening Test, 119
Baseline data, 249
Behavior modification, 199-200, 227
Bill Wilkerson Center, 263
Blissymbolics, 274-275
Blissymbolics Communication Institute, 275
Boehm Test of Basic Concepts, 121
Boel test, 114

C

Cams programs, 254, 259, 260, 266
Carrow Elicited Language Inventory, 124
Case reports, 193-194
Changing objectives, 251
Child groupings, 61-88
Children's Language Processing Inventory, 126
Cleanliness training, 254
Clinical rewards, 199-200, 204
Clustering rehearsal, 240
CNS impaired children,
   language comprehension, 78
   morphological problems, 80-81
   phonological problems, 78-80
   processing problems, 76-78

syntactic problems, 81-84
vocabulary problems, 84-85
Cognitive problems, 49-50
Cognitive training, 226
Communication boards, 275-277
Compilation of individual language data, 193
Constraint variables, 250
Creolization of language, 15-18
Criterion referenced tests, 107-111
Cumulative rehearsal skills, 245

D

Developmental issues, 28-32
Developmental observations, 165
Developmental Sentence Analysis, 128
Development of test items, 100
Direct section boards, 277
Discontinuing objectives, 251
Distinctive feature system, 183-184
Domain-referenced tests, 99, 106-113

E

Early language objectives, 233
Ecological pay-off, 232
Elicitation in treatment, 199-200, 203-204, 208-209, 211-212
Elicitation of linguistic judgments, 177-179, 181
Elicitation for phonological analysis, 182-183
Elicitation of morphology, 199-200, 204
Elicitation of semantics, 188-191
Elicitation of spontaneous sample, 170-172
Eliciting specific structures, 176
Eliminating interfering behaviors, 253
Emotionally disturbed children, 85-88
Encoding boards, 277
Environmental enrichment, 227
Environmentally different children, 63-65

293